Introduction

Welcome to ***"The Vegetarian Athlete's Guide to High-Protein Cooking: 100+ Delicious Recipes "*** Whether you're a seasoned athlete or someone aspiring to reach new fitness heights, this cookbook is tailored to meet your nutritional needs while embracing a plant-based lifestyle.

Contrary to the misconception that vegetarians struggle to consume adequate protein, this book aims to debunk that myth by providing a diverse array of recipes packed with plant-based protein sources. From legumes and grains to nuts and seeds, we've curated a collection of dishes that not only support your athletic endeavors but also tantalize your taste buds.

In these pages, you'll find a fusion of flavors and culinary inspirations from around the world, each recipe meticulously crafted to offer a balance of macronutrients essential for optimizing performance and recovery. Whether you're fueling up for an intense training session or replenishing your body post-workout, these dishes are designed to support your goals.

Beyond the recipes themselves, this book serves as a comprehensive guide for the vegetarian athlete, offering insights into key nutritional principles, meal planning strategies, and tips for maximizing your athletic potential on a plant-based diet. We believe that achieving peak performance isn't just about what you do in the gym or on the field but also about nourishing your body with wholesome, nutrient-dense foods.

As you embark on this culinary journey, we encourage you to explore, experiment, and discover the incredible versatility of plant-based ingredients. Whether you're craving hearty comfort foods, refreshing smoothies, or satisfying snacks, "The Vegetarian Athlete's Guide to High-Protein Cooking" has something for every occasion.

Here's to embracing the power of plants, fueling your athletic ambitions, and savoring every delicious bite along the way. Let's cook, eat, and thrive together!

1. Quinoa salad with black beans and avocado

Ingredients:
- 1 cup quinoa, rinsed
- 2 cups vegetable or chicken broth
- 1 (15 oz) can black beans, rinsed and drained
- 1 avocado, diced
- 1 cup cherry tomatoes, halved
- 1/2 red onion, diced
- 1/4 cup chopped cilantro
- Juice of 1 lime
- 2 tablespoons olive oil
- 1 teaspoon ground cumin
- Salt and pepper to taste

Instructions:

1. Cook the quinoa according to package instructions, using the broth instead of water. Let cool completely.

2. In a large bowl, combine the cooked quinoa, black beans, avocado, cherry tomatoes, red onion, and cilantro.

3. In a small bowl, whisk together the lime juice, olive oil, cumin, and salt and pepper.

4. Pour the dressing over the quinoa mixture and toss gently to combine.

5. Taste and adjust seasoning as needed, adding more lime, salt, pepper, etc. if desired.

6. Serve chilled or at room temperature. Enjoy!

You can add other veggies like diced bell pepper or corn if you'd like. The avocado adds a wonderful creaminess. This makes a tasty, filling vegetarian meal or side dish. Leftovers keep well refrigerated for a few days.

2. Lentil soup with kale

Ingredients:
- 1 cup dried brown or green lentils, rinsed
- 1 tablespoon olive oil
- 1 onion, diced
- 2 carrots, peeled and diced
- 2 celery stalks, diced
- 3 garlic cloves, minced
- 1 teaspoon ground cumin
- 1/2 teaspoon dried thyme
- 6 cups vegetable or chicken broth
- 1 (15 oz) can diced tomatoes
- 2 cups chopped kale leaves, stems removed
- Salt and pepper to taste
- Grated Parmesan cheese for serving (optional)

Instructions:
1. In a large pot or Dutch oven, heat the olive oil over medium-high heat. Add the onion, carrots and celery. Cook for 5 minutes until softened.

2. Add the garlic, cumin and thyme. Cook for 1 minute until fragrant.

3. Add the lentils, broth, and diced tomatoes with their juices. Season with a pinch of salt and pepper.

4. Bring to a boil, then reduce heat and let simmer for 20-25 minutes, until the lentils are tender.

5. Add the chopped kale and let wilt for 2-3 minutes.

6. Taste and adjust seasoning as needed, adding more salt, pepper, herbs or a dash of vinegar if desired.

7. Serve the lentil soup warm, topped with grated Parmesan cheese if desired.

This filling, protein-packed soup is easy to make and perfect for chilly days. You can use vegetable or chicken broth. It's a convenient meal to have for leftovers during the week as well. Enjoy!

3. Chickpea curry with spinach

Ingredients:
- 2 tablespoons olive oil or ghee
- 1 onion, diced
- 3 garlic cloves, minced
- 1 tablespoon grated ginger
- 1 teaspoon garam masala
- 1 teaspoon ground cumin
- 1 teaspoon ground coriander
- 1/4 teaspoon cayenne pepper (or more to taste)
- 1 (15 oz) can diced tomatoes
- 1 (15 oz) can chickpeas, drained and rinsed
- 1 cup vegetable or chicken broth
- 4 cups fresh baby spinach
- Juice of 1/2 lemon
- Salt to taste
- Chopped cilantro for garnish
- Naan or basmati rice for serving

Instructions:

1. In a large skillet or dutch oven, heat the olive oil/ghee over medium heat. Add the onions and cook for 3-4 minutes until translucent.

2. Add the garlic, ginger, garam masala, cumin, coriander and cayenne. Cook for 1 minute until fragrant.

3. Pour in the diced tomatoes with their juices, chickpeas and broth. Season with salt to taste.

4. Bring to a simmer and let cook for 10-12 minutes to allow flavors to meld.

5. Add the fresh spinach and lemon juice. Cook for 2-3 minutes, stirring occasionally, until spinach is wilted.

6. Taste and adjust seasoning as needed, adding more salt, lemon juice or spices. Remove from heat and garnish with chopped cilantro. Serve the chickpea curry over basmati rice or with naan bread on the side.

This vegetarian curry is so flavorful and comforting. The chickpeas provide protein and the spinach adds nutrition. You can easily make it vegan by using vegetable broth. Feel free to add other veggies like potatoes or cauliflower. Adjust the heat level to your taste with the cayenne pepper.

4. Tofu stir-fry with broccoli and bell peppers

Ingredients:
- 14 oz extra-firm tofu, drained and cubed
- 2 tablespoons soy sauce or tamari
- 1 tablespoon rice vinegar
- 1 teaspoon sesame oil
- 2 tablespoons vegetable oil
- 1 red bell pepper, sliced
- 1 yellow or orange bell pepper, sliced
- 4 cups broccoli florets
- 3 cloves garlic, minced
- 1 tablespoon grated ginger
- 2 green onions, sliced
- Cooked brown rice or quinoa, for serving

Sauce:
- 3 tablespoons soy sauce or tamari
- 2 tablespoons rice vinegar
- 1 tablespoon maple syrup or honey
- 1 teaspoon sesame oil
- 1 teaspoon cornstarch
- 1/4 cup water

Instructions:

1. Toss the tofu with the 2 tablespoons soy sauce, 1 tablespoon rice vinegar, and 1 teaspoon sesame oil. Let marinate for 15 minutes.

2. Make the sauce by whisking together the sauce ingredients until cornstarch is dissolved. Set aside.

3. Heat 1 tablespoon oil in a large skillet or wok over high heat. Add the marinated tofu and stir-fry for 5 minutes until lightly browned on all sides. Transfer tofu to a plate.

4. Add the remaining 1 tablespoon oil to the skillet/wok. Add the bell peppers and broccoli and stir-fry for 4 minutes.

5. Add the garlic, ginger and green onions. Cook for 1 minute until fragrant.

6. Return the tofu to the skillet/wok.

7. Whisk the sauce again to recombine and pour it into the vegetable mixture. Toss everything to coat in the sauce.

8. Let cook for 3-4 more minutes, stirring frequently, until sauce thickens slightly and vegetables are crisp-tender. Serve the tofu veggie stir-fry over cooked brown rice or quinoa.

This colorful tofu and veggie stir-fry is packed with plant protein, fiber and nutrients. The tamari (or soy sauce) and sesame oil give it a lovely Asian-inspired flavor. Feel free to add other veggies you enjoy like snap peas, carrots or mushrooms. It makes great leftovers for meal prep too!

5. Greek yogurt parfait with mixed berries and nuts

Ingredients:
- 2 cups plain Greek yogurt
- 1 cup mixed fresh berries (strawberries, blueberries, raspberries, blackberries)
- 2 tablespoons honey or maple syrup
- 1 teaspoon vanilla extract
- 1/4 cup granola or toasted nuts like almonds or pecans
- Mint leaves for garnish (optional)

Instructions:

1. In a small bowl, mix together the Greek yogurt, honey/maple syrup, and vanilla extract until well combined.

2. Use a sharp knife to slice any large berries like strawberries into smaller pieces if desired.

3. In a glass or jar, layer 1/4 of the yogurt mixture, then 1/4 of the mixed berries, repeating the layers until you've used up all the yogurt and berries. End with the berries on top.

4. Optionally, you can create just one large parfait in a bowl rather than individual portions.

5. Sprinkle the granola or toasted nuts over the top of the parfait(s).

6. Garnish with fresh mint leaves if using.

7. Refrigerate for 30 minutes to allow flavors to blend together.

8. When ready to serve, you can add an extra drizzle of honey or maple syrup if desired.

This makes a wonderful breakfast, snack or light dessert! The Greek yogurt provides protein while the berries are full of fiber, vitamins and antioxidants. The nuts add healthy fats and crunch.

You can use any combination of your favorite fresh or frozen berries. Try mixing it up with different yogurt flavors or nut varieties as well. Parfaits are so easy to customize with your favorite ingredients.

6. Black bean and sweet potato tacos

Ingredients:
- 2 medium sweet potatoes, peeled and diced into 1/2-inch cubes
- 2 tablespoons olive oil, divided
- 1 teaspoon chili powder
- 1 teaspoon cumin
- 1 teaspoon paprika
- 1/2 teaspoon garlic powder
- Salt and pepper to taste
- 1 (15 oz) can black beans, drained and rinsed
- 8-10 small corn or flour tortillas
- Toppings: shredded cabbage or lettuce, diced tomatoes, avocado, lime wedges, etc.

Instructions:
1. Preheat oven to 400°F. On a baking sheet, toss the diced sweet potatoes with 1 tablespoon olive oil, chili powder, cumin, paprika, garlic powder and salt and pepper.

2. Roast for 20-25 minutes, tossing halfway, until sweet potatoes are tender and lightly browned.

3. In a skillet over medium-high heat, add the remaining 1 tablespoon olive oil. Add the drained black beans and cook for 2-3 minutes to warm through, smashing some of the beans lightly with a fork to create a chunky texture.

4. Season the black beans with salt, pepper and any additional spices you'd like.

5. Warm the tortillas according to package instructions in the microwave, oven or over a gas burner.

6. To assemble the tacos, place some black beans in each tortilla, top with roasted sweet potatoes and your desired toppings like cabbage, tomatoes, avocado, lime juice, etc.

7. Serve the tacos immediately while the fillings are warm.

These veggie tacos are flavorful, nutritious and easy to make. The roasted sweet potatoes pair beautifully with the earthy black beans. Feel free to add a dollop of sour cream, shredded cheese or other favorite taco toppings.

For a vegan version, use vegan/plant-based tortillas and toppings. You can also turn this into a burrito bowl by serving over rice or greens if preferred. Enjoy!

7. Tempeh lettuce wraps with peanut sauce

Ingredients:
- 8 oz tempeh, crumbled or cubed
- 2 tablespoons soy sauce or tamari
- 2 tablespoons rice vinegar
- 1 tablespoon sesame oil
- 2 carrots, julienned or shredded
- 2 cups shredded red cabbage
- 1/2 cup thinly sliced green onions
- Lettuce leaves for wrapping (Boston, iceberg, butter)

Peanut Sauce:
- 1/4 cup creamy peanut butter
- 2 tablespoons soy sauce or tamari
- 1 tablespoon rice vinegar
- 1 tablespoon maple syrup or honey
- 1-2 teaspoons Sriracha or chili garlic sauce
- 2-3 tablespoons water to thin

Instructions:

1. In a bowl, toss the crumbled/cubed tempeh with the 2 tablespoons soy sauce, 2 tablespoons rice vinegar, and sesame oil. Let marinate for 15-20 minutes.

2. Make the peanut sauce by whisking together the peanut butter, 2 tablespoons soy sauce, 1 tablespoon vinegar, maple syrup, Sriracha and 2-3 tablespoons water to reach a drizzly consistency.

3. Heat a skillet over medium-high heat. Add the marinated tempeh and cook for 5-7 minutes until browned, stirring frequently.

4. Remove tempeh from heat and transfer to a bowl. Add the shredded carrots, cabbage and green onions. Toss to combine.

5. To serve, lay out the lettuce leaves. Spoon the tempeh filling into each lettuce leaf. Drizzle with the peanut sauce.

6. Optionally, you can also add sliced avocado, chopped peanuts, lime wedges or other desired toppings.

These lettuce wraps make such a fresh, flavorful and protein-packed veggie meal! The peanut sauce adds an amazing creamy, savory and slightly sweet note.

You can use whatever lettuce variety you prefer for the wraps. For added crunch, you can stir-fry the carrots and cabbage briefly before mixing with the tempeh if desired.

This recipe is vegan, gluten-free and loaded with plant-based goodness. Perfect for a light lunch or dinner.

8. Edamame and vegetable stir-fry with cashews

Ingredients:
- 3 cloves garlic, minced
- 1 tablespoon grated ginger
- 3 green onions, sliced
- 1/3 cup roasted cashews
- 2 tablespoons soy sauce or tamari
- 1 tablespoon rice vinegar
- 1 teaspoon sesame seeds
- 1 cup shelled edamame (frozen and thawed or fresh)
- 2 tablespoons sesame oil
- 1 red bell pepper, sliced
- 1 cup broccoli florets
- 1 cup sliced mushrooms
- 2 carrots, julienned

Instructions:
1. If using frozen edamame, run under warm water to thaw and drain well. Set aside.

2. Heat sesame oil in a large skillet or wok over medium-high heat.

3. Add the bell pepper, broccoli, mushrooms and carrots. Stir-fry for 4-5 minutes until vegetables are crisp-tender.

4. Add the garlic, ginger and green onions. Cook for 1 minute until fragrant.

5. Add the edamame, cashews, soy sauce and rice vinegar. Toss everything together for 2 more minutes.

6. Remove from heat and transfer stir-fry to a serving dish. Garnish with sesame seeds.

7. Serve over steamed rice or rice noodles if desired.

This veggie-packed stir-fry is loaded with protein, fiber, and an array of vibrant flavors and textures! The edamame provides plant-based protein while the cashews add a delicious crunch.

You can easily customize this dish by swapping in your favorite veggies like snap peas, cabbage, bean sprouts or whatever you have on hand. The ginger, garlic and soy sauce create an irresistible savory-umami sauce that coats everything.

This makes a satisfying vegetarian/vegan main dish or hearty side. The freshness of the edamame and crunch of the cashews really make it special. Enjoy!

9. Spinach and feta stuffed mushrooms

Ingredients:
- 4 oz feta cheese, crumbled
- 1/4 cup panko breadcrumbs
- 2 tablespoons grated parmesan cheese
- 1 egg, lightly beaten
- 1/4 teaspoon dried oregano
- Salt and pepper to taste
- 16-20 medium sized mushrooms (cremini or white)
- 2 tablespoons olive oil, divided
- 1/2 onion, finely diced
- 3 cloves garlic, minced
- 10 oz frozen chopped spinach, thawed and drained of excess moisture

Instructions:

1. Preheat oven to 375°F. Lightly grease a baking dish with non-stick cooking spray.

2. Carefully remove the stems from the mushrooms and finely chop them. Set caps aside.

3. In a skillet, heat 1 tablespoon olive oil over medium heat. Add the chopped mushroom stems and diced onion. Cook for 3 minutes until softened.

4. Add the garlic and cook for 1 minute until fragrant. Remove from heat and let cool slightly.

5. In a bowl, mix together the cooked mushroom stem mixture, thawed and drained spinach, feta, panko, parmesan, egg, oregano and salt and pepper to taste until well combined.

6. Using a spoon, generously stuff the mushroom caps with the spinach and feta filling, mounding it slightly.

7. Arrange the stuffed mushrooms cap-side up in the prepared baking dish. Drizzle or brush the tops with the remaining 1 tablespoon olive oil.

8. Bake for 18-22 minutes until the mushrooms are tender and the tops are lightly browned. Serve the stuffed mushrooms warm. Enjoy!

These bite-sized stuffed mushrooms are SO flavorful! The savory spinach and feta filling is irresistible. They make a tasty vegetarian appetizer or side dish.

For extra flavor, you can sauté the mushroom stems and onion in butter or add a splash of white wine. Different cheeses like goat cheese also work nicely in addition to or instead of feta.

The stuffing can be prepared up to a day in advance and the mushrooms stuffed right before baking. They're an easy but impressive appetizer for any occasion!

10. Protein-packed smoothie
with banana, spinach, and protein powder

Ingredients:
- 1 ripe banana
- 1 cup unsweetened almond milk (or milk of choice)
- 1 cup fresh baby spinach
- 1 scoop (about 25g) vanilla or plain plant-based protein powder
- 1 tablespoon almond butter or peanut butter
- 1 tablespoon ground flaxseed (optional)
- 1 teaspoon honey or maple syrup (optional, if you want it sweeter)
- 1/2 cup ice cubes

Instructions:
1. Add the banana, almond milk, spinach, protein powder, almond butter, flaxseed (if using), honey/maple syrup (if using) and ice cubes to a blender.

2. Blend on high speed until completely smooth and no chunks of spinach remain, about 1 minute.

3. If the smoothie is too thick, add a splash more almond milk to reach your desired consistency.

4. Pour into a glass and enjoy immediately! You can top with extras like sliced banana, granola, etc if desired.

This easy protein smoothie recipe packs in 20-25 grams of plant-based protein from the protein powder to keep you feeling satisfied. The banana makes it creamy and naturally sweet.

The spinach gives it a nutrient boost with iron, fiber and vitamins, while contributing barely any flavor. The healthy fats from the nut butter and optional flaxseed provide lasting energy.

You can use any type of milk, yogurt or juice as the base instead of almond milk. Any nut butter works great or you can omit it. This is a very versatile smoothie - feel free to use your favorite protein powder and adjust ingredients to taste.

It's an amazingly quick and nutritious breakfast or snack! Perfect for replenishing nutrients after a workout too.

11. Eggplant Parmesan with whole wheat pasta

Ingredients:
- 1 (24oz) jar marinara sauce
- 8 oz whole wheat pasta
(spaghetti, linguine, etc)
- 8 oz shredded mozzarella cheese
- 1/4 cup chopped fresh basil
- Olive oil for brushing
- 1 large eggplant, sliced into 1/2-inch rounds
- 1 cup panko breadcrumbs
- 1/2 cup grated parmesan cheese, plus more for topping
- 1 egg, beaten
- 1/4 cup milk

Instructions:

1. Preheat oven to 425°F. Line 2 baking sheets with parchment paper or foil coated with cooking spray.

2. In a shallow bowl, mix together the panko and 1/2 cup parmesan. In another bowl, whisk together the egg and milk.

3. Dip the eggplant rounds into the egg mixture, then into the panko parmesan mixture, coating both sides. Place on the baking sheets.

4. Brush or spray the tops of the breaded eggplant with olive oil. Bake for 18-20 minutes, flipping halfway, until golden brown.

5. Meanwhile, cook the whole wheat pasta according to package instructions until al dente. Drain and set aside.

6. In a 9x13 baking dish, spread 1 cup of the marinara sauce in an even layer. Top with half of the eggplant rounds in a single layer.

7. Pour another 1 cup of sauce over the eggplant and top with half of the mozzarella cheese.

8. Add the remaining eggplant in a single layer, then the remaining sauce and mozzarella cheese.

9. Bake for 20 minutes until hot and the cheese is melted. Remove from oven, top with extra parmesan and basil. Serve the eggplant parmesan over the whole wheat pasta.

This vegetarian eggplant parmesan is so delicious and satisfying! The crispy breaded eggplant pairs perfectly with the marinara and melty cheese. Serving it over whole wheat pasta makes it a hearty, vegetable-packed meal.

For quicker prep, you can grill or air fry the eggplant instead of baking it if desired. Leftovers reheat well for an easy lunch the next day. Enjoy!

12. Cottage cheese pancakes with blueberry compote

Pancake Ingredients:
- 1 cup all-purpose flour
- 2 teaspoons baking powder
- 1/4 teaspoon salt
- 1 cup low-fat cottage cheese
- 2 large eggs
- 1 teaspoon vanilla extract
- 2 tablespoons maple syrup
- Butter or oil for cooking

Blueberry Compote:
- 2 cups fresh or frozen blueberries
- 1/4 cup water
- 2 tablespoons maple syrup
- 1 tablespoon lemon juice
- 1 teaspoon cornstarch
- 1 teaspoon lemon zest

Instructions:

For the Pancakes:
1. In a bowl, whisk together the flour, baking powder and salt.
2. In another bowl, blend the cottage cheese, eggs, vanilla and 2 tbsp maple syrup until smooth.
3. Pour the cottage cheese mixture into the dry ingredients and stir just until combined (do not overmix).
4. Heat a skillet or griddle over medium heat. Brush with butter or oil.
5. For each pancake, pour about 1/4 cup of the batter onto the hot surface. Cook 2-3 minutes until bubbles appear on the surface.
6. Flip and cook 1-2 minutes more until golden brown. Repeat with remaining batter.

For the Blueberry Compote:
1. In a saucepan, combine the blueberries, water, maple syrup and lemon juice.
2. In a small bowl, mix the cornstarch with 2 tbsp water to make a slurry.
3. When the blueberry mixture begins to simmer, stir in the cornstarch slurry.
4. Cook for 2 more minutes, stirring frequently, until thickened.
5. Remove from heat and stir in the lemon zest.

To Serve:
Stack the cottage cheese pancakes and top with the warm blueberry compote. You can also add extra maple syrup, powdered sugar, whipped cream or other desired toppings.

These pancakes have such a wonderful flavor and texture from the cottage cheese. The blueberry compote adds a fresh, vibrant fruity taste.

For extra protein, you can fold some of the cottage cheese right into the pancake batter. Other berry compotes like strawberry or raspberry work nicely too. Enjoy this tasty and satisfying breakfast!

13. Three-bean chili with quinoa

Ingredients:

- 1 tablespoon olive oil
- 1 yellow onion, diced
- 3 cloves garlic, minced
- 2 carrots, diced
- 1 bell pepper, diced
- 2 tablespoons chili powder
- 1 tablespoon cumin
- 1 teaspoon oregano
- 1 cup quinoa
- 1/4 teaspoon cayenne pepper (optional for heat)
- 1 (15oz) can black beans, drained and rinsed
- 1 (15oz) can kidney beans, drained and rinsed
- 1 (15oz) can pinto beans, drained and rinsed
- 1 (28oz) can diced tomatoes
- 1 cup vegetable or chicken broth

- Desired toppings: avocado, cheese, green onions, etc

Instructions:

1. Cook the quinoa according to package instructions. Set aside.

2. In a large pot or dutch oven, heat the olive oil over medium-high heat.

3. Add the onion and sauté for 2-3 minutes until translucent.

4. Add the garlic, carrots, bell pepper and spices (chili powder through cayenne). Cook for 2 more minutes.

5. Pour in the drained beans, diced tomatoes and vegetable broth.

6. Bring the chili to a simmer and let it cook for 15-20 minutes, until slightly thickened.

7. Taste and adjust seasoning as needed, adding more spices, salt and pepper if desired.

8. To serve, scoop the cooked quinoa into bowls and top with the three-bean chili.

9. Add any desired toppings like diced avocado, shredded cheese, green onions, etc.

This veggie-packed three-bean chili is incredibly flavorful, protein-rich and satisfying! The quinoa adds extra heartiness and nutrition.

You can use any combination of canned or cooked dried beans you prefer. Throw in some corn or bell peppers for extra veggies. A dollop of Greek yogurt or sour cream is also a delicious topping.

This recipe makes a big batch that's perfect for meal prep. The chili keeps well refrigerated for several days or you can freeze portions too. So nutritious and delicious!

14. Grilled portobello mushrooms with quinoa salad

For the Mushrooms:
- 4 large portobello mushroom caps
- 2 tablespoons olive oil
- 2 tablespoons balsamic vinegar
- 2 cloves garlic, minced
- 1 teaspoon dried thyme
- Salt and pepper to taste

For the Quinoa Salad:
- 1 cup quinoa, rinsed
- 1 1/2 cups vegetable or chicken broth
- 1 cucumber, diced
- 1 cup cherry tomatoes, halved
- 1/2 red onion, finely diced
- 1/4 cup chopped fresh parsley
- Juice of 1 lemon
- 2 tablespoons olive oil
- Salt and pepper to taste

Instructions:

1. In a bowl, whisk together the olive oil, balsamic vinegar, garlic, thyme and a pinch each of salt and pepper.

2. Remove the stems from the mushroom caps and brush the tops and undersides with the marinade. Let sit for 15-20 minutes.

3. Meanwhile, prepare the quinoa salad. In a saucepan, bring the broth to a boil. Add the rinsed quinoa, cover and simmer for 15-18 minutes until liquid is absorbed.

4. In a bowl, combine the cooked quinoa, cucumber, tomatoes, onion and parsley.

5. Drizzle with lemon juice and olive oil. Season with salt and pepper to taste.

6. Heat a grill or grill pan to medium-high. Grill the mushrooms cap-side down first for 4-5 minutes until grill marks form.

7. Flip and grill for 3-5 more minutes until mushrooms are tender. To serve, place the grilled portobello mushrooms on a bed of the quinoa salad.

The smoky, balsamic-marinated portobellos pair perfectly with the fresh, bright quinoa salad. It's a satisfying yet light vegetarian meal.

For added protein, you can mix in some chickpeas, white beans or feta to the quinoa salad. Other veggies like spinach, zucchini or bell peppers would be delicious additions as well.

The quinoa salad can also be served chilled or at room temperature if preferred. Don't forget a sprinkle of feta or parmesan over the top of the grilled portobellos right before serving. Enjoy!

15. Greek yogurt tzatziki with cucumber and whole wheat pita

Ingredients:
- 2 cups plain Greek yogurt
- 1 English cucumber, grated and drained of excess moisture
- 2 garlic cloves, minced
- 2 tablespoons lemon juice
- 2 tablespoons olive oil
- 1 tablespoon fresh dill, chopped
- 1 tablespoon fresh mint, chopped
- 1 teaspoon red wine vinegar
- 1/2 teaspoon salt
- 1/4 teaspoon black pepper
- Whole wheat pita bread, cut into triangles
- Optional garnishes: sliced cucumber, tomatoes, red onion, olives

Instructions:

1. Grate the cucumber and transfer to a fine mesh strainer. Let sit for 15-20 minutes to drain excess moisture. Then squeeze out any remaining liquid.

2. In a medium bowl, combine the strained grated cucumber with the Greek yogurt, garlic, lemon juice, olive oil, dill, mint, vinegar, salt and pepper.

3. Mix everything together until well incorporated. Taste and adjust seasoning if needed, adding more lemon juice for tang or salt and pepper for flavor.

4. Cover and refrigerate the tzatziki for at least 30 minutes to allow flavors to meld. This can be made up to 2 days in advance.

5. When ready to serve, scoop the tzatziki into a shallow bowl. Use a fork to create grooves and wells for the olive oil to pool in.

6. Garnish with extra chopped dill, mint, sliced cucumbers, tomatoes, red onions and olives if desired.

7. Serve the tzatziki chilled or at room temperature with the whole wheat pita triangles for dipping.

This refreshing Greek yogurt tzatziki makes a wonderful healthy appetizer or snack with the pita bread. It's cool, creamy, tangy and so flavorful.

For extra protein, you can even use the tzatziki as a sauce for grilled chicken or fish. It's also delicious stuffed into a pita sandwich with fresh veggies.

Be sure to drain the grated cucumber fully to prevent excess liquid from thinning out the tzatziki. This simple Mediterranean dip is hard to beat!

16. Veggie burger with avocado and sprouts

Ingredients:
- 1 can (15 oz) black beans, drained and rinsed
- 1/2 cup cooked quinoa
- 1/4 cup finely chopped onion
- 1/4 cup finely chopped bell pepper (any color)
- 2 cloves garlic, minced
- 1 teaspoon ground cumin
- 1 teaspoon smoked paprika
- Salt and pepper to taste
- 1 tablespoon olive oil
- 4 whole grain burger buns
- 1 ripe avocado, sliced
- 1 cup sprouts (such as alfalfa or broccoli sprouts)
- Optional toppings: lettuce, tomato, cheese, mustard, etc.

Instructions:
1. In a large mixing bowl, mash the black beans until they are mostly smooth but still have some texture.

2. Add cooked quinoa, chopped onion, bell pepper, minced garlic, cumin, smoked paprika, salt, and pepper to the bowl. Mix until well combined.

3. Divide the mixture into 4 equal portions and shape each portion into a patty.

4. Heat olive oil in a skillet over medium heat. Once hot, add the veggie patties to the skillet and cook for 4-5 minutes on each side, or until golden brown and heated through.

5. While the patties are cooking, lightly toast the burger buns.

6. To assemble the burgers, place a veggie patty on the bottom half of each bun. Top with sliced avocado and sprouts.

7. Add any additional toppings you desire, such as lettuce, tomato, cheese, or mustard.

8. Cover with the top half of the burger bun and serve immediately.

Enjoy your delicious and nutritious veggie burgers with avocado and sprouts! Feel free to customize the recipe with your favorite toppings and seasonings.

17. Spinach and ricotta stuffed shells

Ingredients:
- 1 box (12 oz) jumbo pasta shells
- 2 cups ricotta cheese
- 1 teaspoon dried oregano
- Salt and pepper to taste
- 2 cups marinara sauce
- Fresh basil leaves for garnish (optional)
- 1 1/2 cups shredded mozzarella cheese, divided
- 1 cup grated Parmesan cheese, divided
- 1 egg
- 2 cups chopped fresh spinach, cooked and drained (frozen spinach can be used as well)
- 2 cloves garlic, minced
- 1 teaspoon dried basil

Instructions:

1. Preheat your oven to 350°F (175°C). Grease a 9x13 inch baking dish with cooking spray or olive oil.

2. Cook the jumbo pasta shells according to the package instructions until they are al dente. Drain and rinse them under cold water to stop the cooking process. Set aside.

3. In a large mixing bowl, combine the ricotta cheese, 1 cup of shredded mozzarella cheese, 1/2 cup of grated Parmesan cheese, egg, chopped spinach, minced garlic, dried basil, dried oregano, salt, and pepper. Mix well until all ingredients are thoroughly combined.

4. Spread a thin layer of marinara sauce on the bottom of the prepared baking dish.

5. Stuff each cooked pasta shell with a generous spoonful of the spinach and ricotta mixture and place them in the baking dish, arranging them in a single layer.

6. Once all the shells are stuffed and placed in the baking dish, spoon the remaining marinara sauce over the top, covering the shells evenly.

7. Sprinkle the remaining shredded mozzarella cheese and grated Parmesan cheese over the top of the shells.

8. Cover the baking dish with aluminum foil and bake in the preheated oven for 25-30 minutes, or until the cheese is melted and bubbly.

9. Remove the foil and bake for an additional 5-10 minutes, or until the cheese is golden brown.

10. Once done, remove from the oven and let it cool slightly before serving. Garnish with fresh basil leaves if desired.

18. Black bean and corn quesadillas

Ingredients:
- 1 can (15 oz) black beans, drained and rinsed
- 1 cup corn kernels (fresh, frozen, or canned)
- 1 cup shredded cheese (cheddar, Monterey Jack, or a blend)
- 1/2 cup diced bell peppers (any color)
- 1/4 cup chopped fresh cilantro
- 1 teaspoon ground cumin
- 1/2 teaspoon chili powder
- Salt and pepper to taste
- 4 large flour tortillas
- Olive oil or cooking spray
- Optional toppings: salsa, sour cream, guacamole, etc.

Instructions:
1. In a mixing bowl, combine black beans, corn, shredded cheese, diced bell peppers, chopped cilantro, ground cumin, chili powder, salt, and pepper. Mix well to combine all the ingredients evenly.

2. Heat a large skillet or griddle over medium heat.

3. Place one flour tortilla on the skillet. Spread a quarter of the bean and corn mixture evenly over half of the tortilla.

4. Fold the other half of the tortilla over the filling, creating a half-moon shape.

5. Cook the quesadilla for 2-3 minutes on each side, or until the tortilla is golden brown and the cheese is melted.

6. Repeat the process with the remaining tortillas and filling.

7. Once cooked, remove the quesadillas from the skillet and let them cool for a minute before slicing them into wedges.

8. Serve hot with your favorite toppings such as salsa, sour cream, or guacamole.

Enjoy these flavorful black bean and corn quesadillas as a quick and satisfying meal or snack!

19. Chia seed pudding with almond milk and berries

Ingredients:

- 1/4 cup chia seeds
- 1 cup almond milk (or any preferred milk)
- 1-2 tablespoons maple syrup or honey (to taste)
- 1/2 teaspoon vanilla extract
- Fresh berries (e.g., strawberries, blueberries, raspberries) for topping
- Optional toppings: sliced almonds, shredded coconut, granola, etc.

Instructions:

1. Combine chia seeds, almond milk, maple syrup (or honey), and vanilla extract in a mixing bowl or jar. Mix thoroughly.
2. Refrigerate the covered mixture for a minimum of 2 hours, or overnight, to allow the chia seeds to absorb the liquid and thicken into a pudding-like consistency. Stir or shake intermittently to prevent clumping.
3. Once the chia seed pudding reaches the desired thickness, give it a final stir.
4. Serve the pudding in individual bowls or jars and garnish with fresh berries.
5. For added flavor and texture, consider including toppings like sliced almonds, shredded coconut, or granola.
6. Delight in the nutritious chia seed pudding with almond milk and berries as a wholesome breakfast, snack, or dessert.

Adjust the sweetness by modifying the amount of maple syrup or honey to suit your taste. Personalize the toppings with your favorite fruits and additional ingredients.

20. Tempeh bacon and avocado toast

Ingredients:
- 1 block of tempeh, sliced thinly
- 2 tablespoons soy sauce or tamari
- 1 tablespoon maple syrup
- 1 tablespoon olive oil
- 1 teaspoon smoked paprika
- 1/2 teaspoon garlic powder
- 1 ripe avocado
- 4 slices of whole grain bread, toasted
- Salt and pepper to taste
- Optional toppings: sliced tomato, red onion, sprouts, etc.

Instructions:
1. In a small bowl, whisk together soy sauce (or tamari), maple syrup, olive oil, smoked paprika, and garlic powder to make the marinade.

2. Place the tempeh slices in a shallow dish or resealable bag and pour the marinade over them. Make sure the tempeh is evenly coated. Let it marinate for at least 15-30 minutes.

3. Heat a non-stick skillet over medium heat. Once hot, add the marinated tempeh slices to the skillet, reserving any excess marinade.

4. Cook the tempeh slices for 2-3 minutes on each side, or until they are crispy and browned. If the skillet becomes dry, you can brush some of the reserved marinade over the tempeh slices while cooking.

5. While the tempeh is cooking, mash the ripe avocado in a small bowl and season with salt and pepper to taste.

6. Once the tempeh slices are done, remove them from the skillet and set aside.

7. To assemble the avocado toast, spread a generous amount of mashed avocado onto each slice of toasted bread.

8. Top the avocado toast with the cooked tempeh bacon slices.

9. Optionally, garnish with additional toppings such as sliced tomato, red onion, or sprouts.

10. Serve the tempeh bacon and avocado toast immediately and enjoy as a delicious and satisfying breakfast, brunch, or snack!

21. Lentil salad with roasted vegetables

Ingredients:
- 1 cup dried green lentils, rinsed and drained
- 3 cups mixed vegetables (such as bell peppers, zucchini, cherry tomatoes, red onion, etc.), chopped into bite-sized pieces
- 2 tablespoons olive oil
- 2 cloves garlic, minced
- 1 teaspoon dried thyme
- Salt and pepper to taste
- 4 cups mixed salad greens (such as spinach, arugula, or lettuce)
- 1/4 cup crumbled feta cheese or goat cheese (optional)
- Balsamic glaze for drizzling (optional)

For the dressing:
- 3 tablespoons extra virgin olive oil
- 2 tablespoons balsamic vinegar
- 1 teaspoon Dijon mustard
- 1 teaspoon honey or maple syrup
- Salt and pepper to taste

Instructions:

1. Preheat your oven to 400°F (200°C).

2. In a large mixing bowl, toss the chopped vegetables with olive oil, minced garlic, dried thyme, salt, and pepper until evenly coated.

3. Spread the seasoned vegetables in a single layer on a baking sheet lined with parchment paper or aluminum foil.

4. Roast the vegetables in the preheated oven for 20-25 minutes, or until they are tender and lightly browned, stirring halfway through the cooking time.

5. While the vegetables are roasting, cook the lentils according to the package instructions until they are tender but still hold their shape. Drain any excess water and set aside to cool.

6. In a small bowl, whisk together the ingredients for the dressing: extra virgin olive oil, balsamic vinegar, Dijon mustard, honey or maple syrup, salt, and pepper.

7. In a large salad bowl, combine the cooked lentils, roasted vegetables, mixed salad greens, and crumbled feta or goat cheese (if using).

8. Drizzle the dressing over the salad and toss gently to combine, ensuring all ingredients are coated evenly.

9. Taste and adjust seasoning with additional salt and pepper if needed. Serve the lentil salad with roasted vegetables immediately, garnished with a drizzle of balsamic glaze if desired.

22. Baked tofu with teriyaki sauce and brown rice

Ingredients:
- 1 block (14 oz) firm or extra firm tofu, pressed and drained
- 1 cup cooked brown rice
- 2 tablespoons soy sauce or tamari
- 2 tablespoons rice vinegar
- 2 tablespoons honey or maple syrup
- 1 clove garlic, minced
- 1 teaspoon grated ginger
- 1 tablespoon cornstarch
- 2 tablespoons water
- Sesame seeds and sliced green onions for garnish (optional)
- Steamed vegetables of your choice (such as broccoli, carrots, or snap peas)

Instructions:
1. Preheat your oven to 400°F (200°C). Line a baking sheet with parchment paper or lightly grease it with oil.

2. Cut the pressed tofu into cubes or rectangles, depending on your preference.

3. In a small bowl, whisk together soy sauce (or tamari), rice vinegar, honey (or maple syrup), minced garlic, and grated ginger to make the teriyaki sauce.

4. In another small bowl, mix cornstarch with water until dissolved to create a slurry.

5. Place the tofu cubes on the prepared baking sheet in a single layer. Brush each tofu piece generously with the teriyaki sauce, reserving some sauce for later.

6. Bake the tofu in the preheated oven for 20-25 minutes, flipping halfway through, until the tofu is golden and slightly crispy.

7. While the tofu is baking, cook the brown rice according to package instructions if you haven't already done so.

8. In a small saucepan, heat the remaining teriyaki sauce over medium heat. Once it starts to simmer, add the cornstarch slurry and whisk continuously until the sauce thickens.

9. Once the tofu is done baking, remove it from the oven and brush with the thickened teriyaki sauce.

10. Serve the baked tofu over cooked brown rice, garnished with sesame seeds and sliced green onions if desired. Serve with steamed vegetables on the side.

23. Caprese salad with fresh mozzarella and basil

Ingredients:
- 2 large ripe tomatoes, sliced
- 1 ball of fresh mozzarella cheese, sliced
- Fresh basil leaves
- Extra virgin olive oil
- Balsamic glaze (optional)
- Salt and pepper to taste

Instructions:

1. Arrange the tomato slices and fresh mozzarella slices on a serving platter, alternating them and slightly overlapping.

2. Tuck fresh basil leaves between the tomato and mozzarella slices.

3. Drizzle extra virgin olive oil over the salad, ensuring it lightly coats the tomatoes and mozzarella.

4. Optionally, drizzle balsamic glaze over the salad for added flavor and a beautiful presentation.

5. Season the salad with salt and pepper to taste.

6. Serve the Caprese salad immediately as a refreshing appetizer or side dish.

Enjoy the vibrant colors and flavors of this classic Caprese salad with fresh mozzarella and basil! It's perfect for showcasing the best of summer produce.

24. Chickpea and vegetable curry

Ingredients:
- 1 can (15 oz) chickpeas, drained and rinsed
- 2 tablespoons vegetable oil
- 1 onion, diced
- 2 cloves garlic, minced
- 1 tablespoon grated ginger
- 1 bell pepper, diced
- 2 carrots, diced
- 1 zucchini, diced
- 1 cup cauliflower florets
- 1 can (14 oz) diced tomatoes
- 1 can (14 oz) coconut milk
- 2 tablespoons curry powder
- 1 teaspoon ground cumin
- 1 teaspoon ground coriander
- 1/2 teaspoon turmeric powder
- Salt and pepper to taste
- Fresh cilantro leaves for garnish (optional)
- Cooked rice or naan bread for serving

Instructions:

1. Heat the vegetable oil in a large skillet or pot over medium heat. Add the diced onion and cook until it becomes translucent, about 3-4 minutes.

2. Add the minced garlic and grated ginger to the skillet and cook for an additional 1-2 minutes, until fragrant.

3. Stir in the diced bell pepper, carrots, zucchini, and cauliflower florets. Cook for 5-6 minutes, stirring occasionally, until the vegetables start to soften.

4. Add the drained chickpeas to the skillet, along with the diced tomatoes and coconut milk. Stir to combine.

5. Sprinkle the curry powder, ground cumin, ground coriander, turmeric powder, salt, and pepper over the vegetable and chickpea mixture. Stir well to evenly distribute the spices.

6. Bring the curry to a simmer, then reduce the heat to low and let it cook for 15-20 minutes, or until the vegetables are tender and the flavors have melded together.

7. Taste and adjust the seasoning as needed, adding more salt and pepper if desired.

8. Serve the chickpea and vegetable curry hot, garnished with fresh cilantro leaves if desired. Enjoy with cooked rice or naan bread.

This hearty and nutritious chickpea and vegetable curry is perfect for a cozy weeknight dinner or meal prep for lunches throughout the week. Feel free to customize the recipe by adding your favorite vegetables or adjusting the spices to suit your taste preferences.

25. Spaghetti squash with marinara sauce and vegan meatballs

Ingredients:
- 1 large spaghetti squash
- 2 cups marinara sauce
- Vegan meatballs
- Olive oil
- Salt and pepper to taste
- Fresh basil leaves for garnish (optional)
- Vegan Parmesan cheese for topping (optional)

Instructions:

1. Halve the spaghetti squash, remove seeds, and roast cut-side down at 400°F (200°C) for 35-45 mins.

2. Warm marinara sauce.

3. Prepare vegan meatballs according to instructions.

4. Scrape cooked spaghetti squash into strands, divide onto plates.

5. Top with warm marinara sauce and vegan meatballs.

6. Garnish with basil leaves and vegan Parmesan cheese if desired.

7. Serve and enjoy!

26. Greek yogurt with honey and sliced almonds

Ingredients:
- 1 cup Greek yogurt
- 1 tablespoon honey (or to taste)
- 2 tablespoons sliced almonds

Instructions:
1. Spoon Greek yogurt into a serving bowl or dish.

2. Drizzle honey over the yogurt, adjusting the amount to your desired sweetness.

3. Sprinkle sliced almonds on top of the yogurt.

4. Serve immediately and enjoy this delicious and nutritious Greek yogurt with honey and sliced almonds!

This makes for a quick and satisfying breakfast, snack, or dessert option that's rich in protein, calcium, and healthy fats. Feel free to customize it with additional toppings such as fresh fruit or granola if desired.

27. Tofu scramble with vegetables and salsa

Ingredients:
- 1 block (14 oz) firm tofu, drained and crumbled
- 1 tablespoon olive oil
- 1 small onion, diced
- 2 cloves garlic, minced
- 1 bell pepper, diced
- 1 cup diced tomatoes
- 2 cups fresh spinach or kale, chopped
- 1 teaspoon ground cumin
- 1/2 teaspoon turmeric powder (for color)
- Salt and pepper to taste
- Salsa for serving
- Optional toppings: avocado slices, chopped cilantro, sliced jalapeños, etc.

Instructions:
1. Heat olive oil in a large skillet over medium heat.

2. Add diced onion and minced garlic to the skillet and sauté until softened and fragrant, about 2-3 minutes.

3. Add diced bell pepper to the skillet and cook for another 2-3 minutes until slightly softened.

4. Add crumbled tofu to the skillet along with ground cumin, turmeric powder, salt, and pepper. Stir to combine and cook for 5-7 minutes, allowing the flavors to meld and the tofu to heat through.

5. Stir in diced tomatoes and chopped spinach or kale. Cook for an additional 2-3 minutes until the vegetables are tender and the tofu is heated through.

6. Taste and adjust seasoning as needed.

7. Serve the tofu scramble hot, topped with salsa and any optional toppings you desire.

8. Enjoy this delicious and satisfying tofu scramble with vegetables and salsa for a nutritious breakfast or brunch!

Feel free to customize the recipe by adding your favorite vegetables or spices to suit your taste preferences.

28. Quinoa stuffed bell peppers

Ingredients:
- 4 large bell peppers (any color)
- 1 cup quinoa, rinsed
- 2 cups vegetable broth or water
- 1 tablespoon olive oil
- 1 small onion, diced
- 2 cloves garlic, minced
- 1 cup diced tomatoes
- 1 cup cooked black beans (canned is fine)
- 1 cup corn kernels (fresh, frozen, or canned)
- 1 teaspoon ground cumin
- 1 teaspoon chili powder
- Salt and pepper to taste
- 1/2 cup shredded cheese (cheddar, mozzarella, or vegan cheese)
- Fresh cilantro leaves for garnish (optional)
- Sliced avocado for serving (optional)
- Salsa or hot sauce for serving (optional)

Instructions:
1. Preheat your oven to 375°F (190°C).

2. Cut the tops off the bell peppers and remove the seeds and membranes from inside.

3. In a medium saucepan, bring vegetable broth or water to a boil. Add quinoa, reduce heat to low, cover, and simmer for 15-20 minutes, or until quinoa is cooked and liquid is absorbed. Remove from heat and let it sit covered for 5 minutes, then fluff with a fork.

4. In a large skillet, heat olive oil over medium heat. Add diced onion and minced garlic, and sauté until softened, about 2-3 minutes.

5. Stir in diced tomatoes, cooked black beans, corn kernels, ground cumin, chili powder, salt, and pepper. Cook for another 2-3 minutes until heated through and well combined.

6. Remove skillet from heat and stir in cooked quinoa until evenly mixed.

7. Stuff each bell pepper with the quinoa mixture, pressing down gently to pack it in.

8. Place stuffed bell peppers in a baking dish. If there's extra filling, you can spoon it around the peppers in the dish.

9. Sprinkle shredded cheese on top of each stuffed bell pepper.

10. Cover the baking dish with aluminum foil and bake in the preheated oven for 25-30 minutes, or until the peppers are tender.

11. Remove the foil and bake for an additional 5-10 minutes, or until the cheese is melted and bubbly.

12. Garnish with fresh cilantro leaves if desired, and serve hot with sliced avocado and salsa or hot sauce on the side.

29. Black bean burgers with avocado and salsa

Ingredients:
- 1 can (15 oz) black beans, drained and rinsed
- 1/2 cup cooked quinoa
- 1/4 cup finely chopped onion
- 1/4 cup finely chopped bell pepper (any color)
- 2 cloves garlic, minced
- 1 teaspoon ground cumin
- 1 teaspoon chili powder
- Salt and pepper to taste
- 1 tablespoon olive oil
- 4 whole grain burger buns
- 1 ripe avocado, sliced
- 1/2 cup salsa (store-bought or homemade)
- Optional toppings: lettuce, tomato, cheese, etc.

Instructions:
1. In a large mixing bowl, mash the black beans until mostly smooth but still chunky.

2. Add cooked quinoa, chopped onion, bell pepper, minced garlic, ground cumin, chili powder, salt, and pepper to the bowl. Mix until well combined.

3. Divide the mixture into 4 equal portions and shape each portion into a patty.

4. Heat olive oil in a skillet over medium heat. Once hot, add the black bean patties to the skillet and cook for 4-5 minutes on each side, or until golden brown and heated through.

5. While the patties are cooking, lightly toast the burger buns.

6. To assemble the burgers, place a black bean patty on the bottom half of each bun. Top with sliced avocado and a spoonful of salsa.

7. Add any additional toppings you desire, such as lettuce, tomato, cheese, or condiments.

8. Cover with the top half of the burger bun and serve immediately.

Enjoy these flavorful and satisfying black bean burgers with creamy avocado and zesty salsa! Feel free to customize the toppings and seasonings to suit your taste preferences.

30. Peanut butter banana protein smoothie

Ingredients:
- 1 ripe banana, peeled and sliced
- 1 tablespoon natural peanut butter (unsweetened)
- 1 scoop of your favorite protein powder (vanilla or chocolate flavored)
- 1 cup unsweetened almond milk (or any milk of your choice)
- 1/2 cup plain Greek yogurt (optional, for added creaminess)
- 1 tablespoon honey or maple syrup (optional, for added sweetness)
- Ice cubes (optional, for a colder smoothie)

Instructions:
1. Place all the ingredients in a blender.

2. Blend on high speed until smooth and creamy.

3. Taste the smoothie and adjust sweetness if necessary by adding more honey or maple syrup.

4. If you prefer a thicker consistency, you can add more banana or a handful of ice cubes and blend again until desired consistency is reached.

5. Pour the smoothie into a glass and enjoy immediately.

This peanut butter banana protein smoothie is perfect for a quick and nutritious breakfast or post-workout snack. Feel free to customize it by adding your favorite ingredients such as spinach, cocoa powder, or chia seeds for extra nutrition!

31. Spinach and mushroom omelette with feta cheese

Ingredients:
- 3 large eggs
- 1 tablespoon butter or olive oil
- 1 cup sliced mushrooms
- 1 cup fresh spinach leaves, roughly chopped
- 1/4 cup crumbled feta cheese
- Salt and pepper to taste
- Fresh herbs for garnish (optional)

Instructions:

1. In a small bowl, beat the eggs until well mixed. Season with salt and pepper to taste.

2. Heat the butter or olive oil in a non-stick skillet over medium heat.

3. Add the sliced mushrooms to the skillet and cook for 3-4 minutes until they start to soften.

4. Add the chopped spinach to the skillet and cook for another 1-2 minutes until wilted.

5. Pour the beaten eggs evenly over the mushrooms and spinach in the skillet.

6. Allow the eggs to cook undisturbed for 2-3 minutes until the edges start to set.

7. Using a spatula, gently lift the edges of the omelette and tilt the skillet to allow the uncooked eggs to flow underneath.

8. Once the eggs are mostly set but still slightly runny on top, sprinkle the crumbled feta cheese evenly over one half of the omelette.

9. Carefully fold the other half of the omelette over the cheese to form a half-moon shape.

10. Cook for another 1-2 minutes until the cheese is melted and the omelette is cooked through.

11. Slide the omelette onto a plate and garnish with fresh herbs if desired. Serve hot and enjoy your delicious spinach and mushroom omelette with feta cheese!

This omelette is perfect for a quick and satisfying breakfast or brunch. Feel free to customize it by adding other ingredients such as diced onions, bell peppers, or tomatoes to suit your taste preferences.

32. Lentil and vegetable stir-fry

Ingredients:
- 1 cup dried green or brown lentils, rinsed
- 2 cups water or vegetable broth
- 2 tablespoons soy sauce or tamari
- 1 tablespoon rice vinegar
- 1 tablespoon sesame oil
- 2 cloves garlic, minced
- 1 teaspoon grated ginger
- 1 onion, thinly sliced
- 2 cups mixed vegetables (such as bell peppers, carrots, broccoli, snap peas)
- Cooked rice or quinoa for serving
- Optional garnishes: sliced green onions, sesame seeds, cilantro

Instructions:
1. In a saucepan, combine lentils and water or vegetable broth. Bring to a boil, then reduce heat to low and simmer, covered, for 20-25 minutes, or until lentils are tender but still hold their shape. Drain any excess liquid and set aside.

2. In a small bowl, whisk together soy sauce or tamari, rice vinegar, and sesame oil to make the stir-fry sauce. Set aside.

3. Heat a large skillet or wok over medium-high heat. Add a bit of oil if needed.

4. Add minced garlic and grated ginger to the skillet and sauté for 1-2 minutes until fragrant.

5. Add sliced onion to the skillet and cook for 2-3 minutes until softened.

6. Add mixed vegetables to the skillet and stir-fry for 5-7 minutes until they are crisp-tender.

7. Stir in cooked lentils and the prepared stir-fry sauce. Cook for an additional 2-3 minutes until everything is heated through and well coated in the sauce.

8. Remove from heat and serve the lentil and vegetable stir-fry over cooked rice or quinoa.

9. Garnish with sliced green onions, sesame seeds, and cilantro if desired. Serve hot and enjoy this flavorful and nutritious lentil and vegetable stir-fry!

Feel free to customize the recipe with your favorite vegetables and add extra spices or chili flakes for a bit of heat.

33. Greek yogurt with granola and mixed berries

Ingredients:
- 1 cup Greek yogurt
- 1/4 cup granola (store-bought or homemade)
- 1/2 cup mixed berries (such as strawberries, blueberries, raspberries)
- Honey or maple syrup (optional, for sweetness)
- Fresh mint leaves for garnish (optional)

Instructions:
1. Spoon Greek yogurt into a serving bowl or dish.

2. Sprinkle granola evenly over the yogurt.

3. Wash and prepare the mixed berries as needed, then scatter them over the granola.

4. Drizzle honey or maple syrup over the top if desired, for added sweetness.

5. Garnish with fresh mint leaves for a burst of freshness and color.

6. Serve immediately and enjoy this delicious and nutritious Greek yogurt with granola and mixed berries!

This breakfast or snack is not only tasty but also packed with protein, fiber, and antioxidants. Feel free to customize it by adding nuts, seeds, or other fruits according to your preference.

34. Tempeh tacos with mango salsa

Ingredients:
For the Tempeh:
- 1 package (8 oz) tempeh, crumbled
- 2 tablespoons olive oil
- 2 cloves garlic, minced
- 1 teaspoon ground cumin
- 1 teaspoon chili powder
- Salt and pepper to taste
- 8 small corn or flour tortillas

For the Mango Salsa:
- 1 ripe mango, diced
- 1/2 red onion, finely chopped
- 1 jalapeño pepper, seeded and minced
- 1/4 cup chopped fresh cilantro
- Juice of 1 lime
- Salt to taste

Optional Toppings:
- Shredded lettuce or cabbage
- Sliced avocado
- Sour cream or dairy-free yogurt
- Crumbled feta cheese or vegan cheese
- Lime wedges for serving

Instructions:
1. In a skillet, heat olive oil over medium heat. Add minced garlic and cook for about 1 minute until fragrant.

2. Add crumbled tempeh to the skillet and sprinkle with ground cumin, chili powder, salt, and pepper. Cook for 8-10 minutes, stirring occasionally, until tempeh is browned and slightly crispy.

3. While the tempeh is cooking, prepare the mango salsa. In a bowl, combine diced mango, finely chopped red onion, minced jalapeño pepper, chopped cilantro, lime juice, and salt. Mix well and set aside.

4. Warm the tortillas according to package instructions or preference.

5. To assemble the tacos, spoon the cooked tempeh onto each tortilla.

6. Top with mango salsa and any optional toppings you desire, such as shredded lettuce or cabbage, sliced avocado, sour cream or dairy-free yogurt, and crumbled feta cheese or vegan cheese.

7. Serve the tempeh tacos immediately, with lime wedges on the side for squeezing.

Enjoy the delicious combination of savory tempeh and sweet mango salsa in these flavorful tacos! They're perfect for a quick and satisfying meal any day of the week.

35. Egg salad sandwich with whole wheat bread

Ingredients:
- 4 hard-boiled eggs, peeled and chopped
- 2 tablespoons mayonnaise
- 1 tablespoon Dijon mustard
- 1 tablespoon chopped fresh chives (optional)
- Salt and pepper to taste
- 8 slices whole wheat bread
- Lettuce leaves (optional)
- Sliced tomato (optional)
- Sliced cucumber (optional)
- Pickles (optional)

Instructions:
1. In a mixing bowl, combine the chopped hard-boiled eggs, mayonnaise, Dijon mustard, chopped chives (if using), salt, and pepper. Mix well until all ingredients are evenly combined.

2. Taste the egg salad and adjust seasoning if needed, adding more salt, pepper, or mustard according to your preference.

3. Lay out the slices of whole wheat bread on a clean surface.

4. Spread a generous amount of the egg salad onto half of the bread slices.

5. If desired, layer lettuce leaves, sliced tomato, sliced cucumber, or pickles on top of the egg salad.

6. Top with the remaining slices of bread to form sandwiches.

7. Press down gently on each sandwich to secure the filling.

8. Using a sharp knife, cut each sandwich in half diagonally or straight across.

9. Serve the egg salad sandwiches immediately, or wrap them tightly in plastic wrap or parchment paper for later.

Enjoy these delicious and satisfying egg salad sandwiches with whole wheat bread for a tasty and nutritious meal! They're perfect for lunch, picnics, or a quick and easy dinner option.

36. Tofu and vegetable kebabs with quinoa

Ingredients:
For the Kebabs:
- 1 block (14 oz) firm tofu,
pressed and cubed
- 1 bell pepper, cut into chunks
- 1 zucchini, sliced into rounds
- 1 red onion, cut into chunks
- Cherry tomatoes
- Wooden or metal skewers

Instructions:
1. If using wooden skewers, soak them in
 water for at least 30 minutes to prevent burning.

For the Marinade:
- 1/4 cup soy sauce or tamari
- 2 tablespoons olive oil
- 2 tablespoons maple syrup or honey
- 2 cloves garlic, minced
- 1 teaspoon grated ginger
- 1 teaspoon ground cumin
- Salt and pepper to taste

For Serving:
- Cooked quinoa

2. In a mixing bowl, whisk together the ingredients for the marinade: soy sauce or tamari, olive oil, maple syrup or honey, minced garlic, grated ginger, ground cumin, salt, and pepper.

3. Place the cubed tofu, bell pepper chunks, zucchini slices, red onion chunks, and cherry tomatoes in a large resealable bag or shallow dish. Pour the marinade over the tofu and vegetables, ensuring they are well coated. Marinate in the refrigerator for at least 30 minutes, or up to 2 hours.

4. Preheat your grill or grill pan over medium-high heat.

5. Thread the marinated tofu and vegetables onto skewers, alternating the ingredients.

6. Grill the kebabs for 8-10 minutes, turning occasionally, until the tofu is lightly charred and the vegetables are tender.

7. While the kebabs are cooking, prepare the quinoa according to package instructions.

8. Serve the tofu and vegetable kebabs hot, alongside cooked quinoa.

9. Enjoy this flavorful and nutritious meal!

These tofu and vegetable kebabs with quinoa are perfect for a healthy and satisfying lunch or dinner. Feel free to customize the vegetables and marinade to suit your taste preferences!

37. Protein-packed oatmeal with almond butter and bananas

Ingredients:
- 1/2 cup old-fashioned rolled oats
- 1 cup unsweetened almond milk (or any milk of your choice)
- 1 tablespoon almond butter
- 1 ripe banana, sliced
- 1 scoop vanilla protein powder
- 1 tablespoon honey or maple syrup (optional, for added sweetness)
- Pinch of cinnamon (optional)
- Chopped nuts or seeds for garnish (optional)

Instructions:
1. In a small saucepan, combine the rolled oats and almond milk. Bring to a gentle boil over medium heat, then reduce the heat to low and simmer for 3-5 minutes, stirring occasionally, until the oats are cooked to your desired consistency.

2. Stir in the almond butter until it's fully incorporated into the oatmeal.

3. Add the sliced banana to the oatmeal and stir gently to combine.

4. If using, stir in the vanilla protein powder until smooth and well mixed.

5. Taste the oatmeal and adjust sweetness if desired by adding honey or maple syrup.

6. If using, sprinkle a pinch of cinnamon over the oatmeal and stir to combine.

7. Remove the oatmeal from heat and transfer it to a serving bowl.

8. Garnish with chopped nuts or seeds if desired.

9. Serve hot and enjoy this protein-packed oatmeal with almond butter and bananas!

This oatmeal is not only delicious but also provides a good balance of complex carbohydrates, protein, and healthy fats to keep you energized and satisfied throughout the morning. Feel free to customize it with your favorite toppings such as shredded coconut, berries, or a drizzle of additional almond butter.

38. Black bean and corn salad with lime vinaigrette

Ingredients:
For the Salad:
- 1 can (15 oz) black beans, drained and rinsed
- 1 cup corn kernels (fresh, canned, or thawed if frozen)
- 1 red bell pepper, diced
- 1/2 red onion, finely chopped
- 1/4 cup chopped fresh cilantro
- 1 avocado, diced (optional)

For the Lime Vinaigrette:
- 2 tablespoons olive oil
- Juice of 2 limes
- 1 teaspoon honey or maple syrup
- 1 clove garlic, minced
- 1/2 teaspoon ground cumin
- Salt and pepper to taste

Instructions:

1. In a large mixing bowl, combine the black beans, corn kernels, diced red bell pepper, finely chopped red onion, and chopped fresh cilantro. If using avocado, add it to the bowl as well.

2. In a small bowl, whisk together the ingredients for the lime vinaigrette: olive oil, lime juice, honey or maple syrup, minced garlic, ground cumin, salt, and pepper.

3. Pour the lime vinaigrette over the black bean and corn salad and toss gently to coat all the ingredients evenly.

4. Taste the salad and adjust seasoning if necessary, adding more salt, pepper, or lime juice to taste.

5. Cover the salad and refrigerate for at least 30 minutes to allow the flavors to meld together.

6. Before serving, give the salad a final toss and adjust seasoning if needed.

7. Serve chilled as a side dish or a light meal.

Enjoy this vibrant and flavorful black bean and corn salad with lime vinaigrette! It's perfect for picnics, barbecues, or as a refreshing side dish any time of the year.

39. Veggie stir-fry with tofu and cashews

Ingredients:
- 1 block (14 oz) firm tofu, pressed and cubed
- 2 tablespoons soy sauce or tamari
- 1 tablespoon sesame oil
- 2 tablespoons vegetable oil
- 2 cloves garlic, minced
- 1 tablespoon grated ginger
- 1 onion, sliced
- 2 bell peppers, sliced
- 1 cup broccoli florets
- 1 cup snow peas, trimmed
- 1/2 cup unsalted cashews
- Cooked rice or noodles for serving

Stir-Fry Sauce:
- 1/4 cup soy sauce or tamari
- 2 tablespoons rice vinegar
- 1 tablespoon maple syrup or honey
- 1 teaspoon cornstarch
- Red pepper flakes (optional, for heat)

Instructions:

1. In a small bowl, mix together the soy sauce or tamari, sesame oil, and cubed tofu. Set aside to marinate while you prepare the vegetables.

2. In another small bowl, whisk together the ingredients for the stir-fry sauce: soy sauce or tamari, rice vinegar, maple syrup or honey, cornstarch, and red pepper flakes if using. Set aside.

3. Heat vegetable oil in a large skillet or wok over medium-high heat. Add minced garlic and grated ginger, and cook for 1 minute until fragrant.

4. Add sliced onion to the skillet and stir-fry for 2-3 minutes until softened.

5. Add sliced bell peppers, broccoli florets, and snow peas to the skillet. Stir-fry for another 5-6 minutes until the vegetables are tender-crisp.

6. Push the vegetables to one side of the skillet and add the marinated tofu to the other side. Cook for 4-5 minutes, stirring occasionally, until the tofu is golden brown on all sides.

7. Pour the stir-fry sauce over the vegetables and tofu in the skillet. Stir well to coat everything evenly in the sauce.

8. Add unsalted cashews to the skillet and toss to combine. Cook for an additional 1-2 minutes until the sauce has thickened slightly. Remove from heat and serve the veggie stir-fry with tofu and cashews hot, over cooked rice or noodles.

Enjoy this flavorful and nutritious veggie stir-fry with tofu and cashews as a delicious and satisfying meal! Feel free to customize it with your favorite vegetables and adjust the seasonings to suit your taste preferences.

40. Greek yogurt ranch dip with vegetable crudites

Ingredients:
- 1 cup Greek yogurt
- 2 tablespoons mayonnaise
- 1 tablespoon lemon juice
- 1 clove garlic, minced
- 1 teaspoon onion powder
- 1 teaspoon dried dill
- 1 teaspoon dried parsley
- 1/2 teaspoon dried chives
- Salt and pepper to taste
- Assorted vegetable crudites (carrot sticks, cucumber slices, bell pepper strips, cherry tomatoes, etc.)

Instructions:
1. In a mixing bowl, combine Greek yogurt, mayonnaise, lemon juice, minced garlic, onion powder, dried dill, dried parsley, dried chives, salt, and pepper. Mix well until all ingredients are fully incorporated.

2. Taste the dip and adjust seasoning if necessary, adding more salt, pepper, or lemon juice to taste.

3. Cover the bowl and refrigerate the dip for at least 30 minutes to allow the flavors to meld together.

4. Before serving, give the dip a final stir and transfer it to a serving bowl.

5. Arrange the assorted vegetable crudites on a platter or serving tray alongside the Greek yogurt ranch dip.

6. Serve the dip and vegetable crudites together as a tasty and nutritious snack or appetizer.

Enjoy this creamy and flavorful Greek yogurt ranch dip with crunchy vegetable crudites for a refreshing and satisfying snack or appetizer! Feel free to customize the dip with additional herbs or spices according to your taste preferences.

41. Chickpea and spinach curry with brown rice

Ingredients:
For the Curry:
- 1 tablespoon vegetable oil
- 1 onion, finely chopped
- 2 cloves garlic, minced
- 1 tablespoon grated ginger
- 1 tablespoon curry powder
- 1 teaspoon ground cumin
- 1 teaspoon ground coriander
- 1/2 teaspoon turmeric powder

- 1/4 teaspoon cayenne pepper (optional, for heat)
- 1 can (15 oz) chickpeas, drained and rinsed
- 1 can (14 oz) diced tomatoes
- 1 can (14 oz) coconut milk
- 4 cups fresh spinach leaves, roughly chopped
- Salt and pepper to taste
- Fresh cilantro leaves for garnish (optional)

For Serving:
- Cooked brown rice

Instructions:
1. Heat vegetable oil in a large skillet or pot over medium heat. Add finely chopped onion and cook for 5-6 minutes until softened and translucent.

2. Add minced garlic and grated ginger to the skillet and cook for 1-2 minutes until fragrant.

3. Stir in curry powder, ground cumin, ground coriander, turmeric powder, and cayenne pepper if using. Cook for another minute until the spices are toasted and aromatic.

4. Add drained and rinsed chickpeas, diced tomatoes (with their juices), and coconut milk to the skillet. Stir well to combine.

5. Bring the curry to a simmer and let it cook for 10-15 minutes, stirring occasionally, until the flavors meld together and the sauce thickens slightly.

6. Stir in roughly chopped spinach leaves and cook for another 3-5 minutes until the spinach wilts.

7. Taste the curry and adjust seasoning with salt and pepper as needed.

8. Remove the skillet from heat and garnish the chickpea and spinach curry with fresh cilantro leaves if desired. Serve hot over cooked brown rice.

Enjoy this hearty and flavorful chickpea and spinach curry with brown rice for a satisfying and nutritious meal! Feel free to adjust the spices and add extra vegetables according to your taste preferences.

42. Lentil loaf with mashed sweet potatoes

Lentil Loaf:
- Cook lentils until tender.

- Sauté onion, garlic, carrots, and celery.

- Add spices, tomato paste, soy sauce, salt, pepper.

- Combine cooked lentils, sautéed vegetables, breadcrumbs, and flax eggs.

- Press mixture into a greased loaf pan and bake at 375°F (190°C) for 40-45 minutes.

Mashed Sweet Potatoes:
- Boil cubed sweet potatoes until tender.

- Mash with butter (or vegan butter), salt, and pepper.

Serve lentil loaf slices with mashed sweet potatoes. Enjoy!

43. Tofu and vegetable spring rolls with peanut dipping sauce

Ingredients:
For the Spring Rolls:
- Rice paper wrappers
- Firm tofu, sliced into strips
- Carrots, julienned
- Cucumber, julienned
- Bell peppers, thinly sliced
- Lettuce leaves
- Fresh herbs
(such as mint, basil, or cilantro)
- Rice vermicelli noodles, cooked
according to package instructions (optional)

For the Peanut Dipping Sauce:
- 1/4 cup creamy peanut butter
- 2 tablespoons soy sauce or tamari
- 1 tablespoon rice vinegar
- 1 tablespoon maple syrup or honey
- 1 clove garlic, minced
- 1 teaspoon grated ginger
- Water, as needed to thin out the sauce

Instructions:
For the Peanut Dipping Sauce:
1. In a small bowl, whisk together peanut butter, soy sauce or tamari, rice vinegar, maple syrup or honey, minced garlic, and grated ginger until smooth.
2. If the sauce is too thick, add water, a little at a time, until you reach your desired consistency. Set aside.

For the Spring Rolls:

1. Prepare all your filling ingredients and have them ready for assembly.

2. Fill a large shallow dish with warm water. Dip one rice paper wrapper into the water and let it soften for about 15-20 seconds until pliable.

3. Place the softened rice paper wrapper on a clean surface. Arrange a few slices of tofu, julienned carrots, cucumber, bell peppers, lettuce leaves, fresh herbs, and cooked rice vermicelli noodles (if using) in the center of the wrapper.

4. Fold the bottom of the wrapper over the filling, then fold in the sides, and roll tightly to enclose the filling like a burrito.

5. Repeat with the remaining rice paper wrappers and filling ingredients.

6. Serve the tofu and vegetable spring rolls with the peanut dipping sauce on the side for dipping.

Enjoy these fresh and flavorful tofu and vegetable spring rolls with peanut dipping sauce as a delicious appetizer or light meal! Feel free to customize the filling with your favorite vegetables and herbs.

44. Quinoa tabbouleh with cucumber and tomatoes

Ingredients:
- 1 cup quinoa, rinsed
- 2 cups water or vegetable broth
- 1 cucumber, diced
- 2 tomatoes, diced
- 1/2 red onion, finely chopped
- 1/4 cup fresh parsley, chopped
- 1/4 cup fresh mint leaves, chopped
- 1/4 cup lemon juice
- 2 tablespoons olive oil
- Salt and pepper to taste

Instructions:

1. In a saucepan, combine quinoa and water or vegetable broth. Bring to a boil, then reduce heat to low, cover, and simmer for 15-20 minutes, or until quinoa is cooked and liquid is absorbed. Remove from heat and let it cool.

2. In a large mixing bowl, combine the cooked quinoa, diced cucumber, diced tomatoes, finely chopped red onion, chopped fresh parsley, and chopped fresh mint leaves.

3. In a small bowl, whisk together lemon juice, olive oil, salt, and pepper to make the dressing.

4. Pour the dressing over the quinoa tabbouleh mixture and toss until well combined.

5. Taste and adjust seasoning if needed, adding more salt, pepper, or lemon juice according to your preference.

6. Cover and refrigerate the quinoa tabbouleh for at least 30 minutes to allow the flavors to meld together.

7. Serve chilled as a refreshing salad or side dish.

Enjoy this light and flavorful quinoa tabbouleh with cucumber and tomatoes as a nutritious addition to your meal! It's perfect for picnics, potlucks, or as a simple side dish any time of the year.

45. Greek yogurt with sliced peaches and almonds

Ingredients:
- 1 cup Greek yogurt
- 1 ripe peach, sliced
- 2 tablespoons sliced almonds
- Honey or maple syrup (optional, for added sweetness)

Instructions:
1. Spoon Greek yogurt into a serving bowl or dish.

2. Arrange sliced peaches on top of the Greek yogurt.

3. Sprinkle sliced almonds over the peaches.

4. If desired, drizzle honey or maple syrup over the top for added sweetness.

5. Serve immediately and enjoy this delightful Greek yogurt with sliced peaches and almonds!

This combination of creamy Greek yogurt, sweet peaches, and crunchy almonds makes for a delicious and satisfying breakfast or snack. Feel free to customize it by adding other fruits or nuts according to your taste preferences.

46. Tempeh bacon BLT wrap

Ingredients:
- 4 slices of tempeh bacon
- 4 large lettuce leaves
- 1 large tomato, thinly sliced
- 1 avocado, sliced
- 4 whole wheat or gluten-free wraps

For the Sauce:
- 1/4 cup mayonnaise (or vegan mayo)
- 1 tablespoon Dijon mustard
- 1 tablespoon maple syrup
- 1 teaspoon smoked paprika
- Salt and pepper to taste

Instructions:
1. Cook the tempeh bacon according to package instructions until crispy.

2. In a small bowl, mix together mayonnaise, Dijon mustard, maple syrup, smoked paprika, salt, and pepper to make the sauce.

3. Lay out the wraps on a clean surface.

4. Spread a generous amount of the sauce over each wrap.

5. Place a lettuce leaf on each wrap, followed by slices of tomato and avocado.

6. Top with cooked tempeh bacon slices.

7. Roll up the wraps tightly, folding in the sides as you go.

8. Slice each wrap in half diagonally, if desired.

9. Serve immediately and enjoy your delicious tempeh bacon BLT wraps!

These wraps are perfect for a quick and satisfying lunch or dinner. The combination of smoky tempeh bacon, crispy lettuce, juicy tomatoes, creamy avocado, and flavorful sauce is sure to please your taste buds!

47. Lentil and vegetable soup

Ingredients:
- 1 cup dry green or brown lentils, rinsed
- 6 cups vegetable broth
- 1 tablespoon olive oil
- 1 onion, chopped
- 2 carrots, diced
- 2 celery stalks, diced
- 2 cloves garlic, minced
- 1 can (14 oz) diced tomatoes
- 2 cups chopped vegetables (such as bell peppers, zucchini, or spinach)
- 1 teaspoon dried thyme
- 1 teaspoon dried oregano
- Salt and pepper to taste
- Fresh parsley for garnish (optional)

Instructions:

1. In a large pot, heat olive oil over medium heat. Add chopped onion, carrots, and celery. Cook for 5-7 minutes until vegetables are softened.

2. Add minced garlic to the pot and cook for another minute until fragrant.

3. Stir in dry lentils, diced tomatoes (with their juices), chopped vegetables, dried thyme, dried oregano, salt, and pepper.

4. Pour in vegetable broth and bring the soup to a boil.

5. Reduce heat to low, cover, and simmer for 20-25 minutes, or until lentils and vegetables are tender.

6. Taste the soup and adjust seasoning if needed, adding more salt and pepper as desired.

7. Serve hot, garnished with fresh parsley if desired.

Enjoy this nourishing and comforting lentil and vegetable soup as a satisfying meal on its own or with a side of crusty bread for dipping. It's perfect for chilly days and makes great leftovers for lunch the next day!

48. Tofu and broccoli stir-fry with sesame seeds

Ingredients:
- 1 block (14 oz) firm tofu, pressed and cubed
- 2 tablespoons soy sauce or tamari
- 1 tablespoon sesame oil
- 1 tablespoon vegetable oil
- 2 cloves garlic, minced
- 1 tablespoon grated ginger
- 1 head broccoli, cut into florets
- 2 tablespoons sesame seeds
- Cooked rice or noodles for serving

Instructions:
1. In a small bowl, mix together soy sauce or tamari, and sesame oil. Add cubed tofu to the bowl and gently toss to coat. Let it marinate for about 10-15 minutes.

2. Heat vegetable oil in a large skillet or wok over medium-high heat. Add minced garlic and grated ginger, and cook for 1 minute until fragrant.

3. Add marinated tofu cubes to the skillet in a single layer. Cook for 3-4 minutes on each side until golden brown and crispy. Remove tofu from the skillet and set aside.

4. In the same skillet, add broccoli florets and stir-fry for 4-5 minutes until tender-crisp.

5. Return the cooked tofu to the skillet with the broccoli. Sprinkle sesame seeds over the tofu and broccoli, and stir-fry for another 1-2 minutes until everything is heated through.

6. Serve the tofu and broccoli stir-fry hot, over cooked rice or noodles.

Enjoy this delicious and nutritious tofu and broccoli stir-fry with sesame seeds as a quick and satisfying meal! Feel free to add extra vegetables or customize the sauce according to your taste preferences.

49. Protein pancakes with Greek yogurt and berries

Ingredients:
- 1 cup rolled oats
- 1 ripe banana
- 1/2 cup Greek yogurt
- 2 eggs
- 1 teaspoon vanilla extract
- 1 teaspoon baking powder
- Pinch of salt
- Butter or oil for cooking
- Fresh berries (such as strawberries, blueberries, or raspberries) for serving
- Maple syrup or honey for drizzling (optional)

Instructions:

1. In a blender or food processor, combine rolled oats, ripe banana, Greek yogurt, eggs, vanilla extract, baking powder, and a pinch of salt. Blend until smooth and well combined.

2. Heat a non-stick skillet or griddle over medium heat. Add a small amount of butter or oil to coat the surface.

3. Pour the pancake batter onto the skillet to form pancakes of your desired size.

4. Cook the pancakes for 2-3 minutes on one side, or until bubbles start to form on the surface. Flip the pancakes and cook for an additional 1-2 minutes on the other side, or until golden brown and cooked through.

5. Repeat with the remaining batter, adding more butter or oil to the skillet as needed.

6. Serve the protein pancakes warm, topped with a dollop of Greek yogurt and fresh berries.

7. If desired, drizzle maple syrup or honey over the pancakes for added sweetness.

Enjoy these protein-packed pancakes with creamy Greek yogurt and juicy berries for a delicious and nutritious breakfast or brunch option! They're sure to satisfy your cravings and keep you energized throughout the morning.

50. Black bean and corn stuffed peppers

Ingredients:
- 4 large bell peppers, any color
- 1 can (15 oz) black beans, drained and rinsed
- 1 cup corn kernels (fresh, canned, or thawed if frozen)
- 1 small onion, diced
- 2 cloves garlic, minced
- 1 teaspoon ground cumin
- 1 teaspoon chili powder
- Salt and pepper to taste
- 1 cup cooked quinoa or rice
- 1 cup shredded cheese (cheddar, Monterey Jack, or Mexican blend)
- Chopped fresh cilantro for garnish (optional)
- Salsa, avocado, sour cream, or Greek yogurt for serving (optional)

Instructions:

1. Preheat your oven to 375°F (190°C). Grease a baking dish large enough to fit the peppers.

2. Cut the tops off the bell peppers and remove the seeds and membranes. Arrange the peppers upright in the prepared baking dish.

3. In a large skillet, heat a little oil over medium heat. Add diced onion and minced garlic, and cook until softened, about 3-4 minutes.

4. Add black beans, corn kernels, ground cumin, chili powder, salt, and pepper to the skillet. Cook for another 3-4 minutes until heated through and well combined.

5. Remove the skillet from heat and stir in cooked quinoa or rice.

6. Stuff the mixture evenly into the hollowed-out bell peppers, pressing down gently to pack the filling.

7. Sprinkle shredded cheese over the top of each stuffed pepper.

8. Cover the baking dish with foil and bake in the preheated oven for 25-30 minutes, or until the peppers are tender and the cheese is melted and bubbly.

9. Remove the foil and bake for an additional 5 minutes to lightly brown the cheese, if desired.

10. Garnish with chopped fresh cilantro, if using, and serve the black bean and corn stuffed peppers hot. Enjoy with your favorite toppings such as salsa, avocado, sour cream, or Greek yogurt.

These black bean and corn stuffed peppers are a delicious and satisfying vegetarian meal that's easy to make and full of flavor. They're perfect for a weeknight dinner or for entertaining guests!

51. Chickpea salad with cucumbers and tomatoes

Ingredients:
- 1 can (15 oz) chickpeas, drained and rinsed
- 1 cucumber, diced
- 1 cup cherry tomatoes, halved
- 1/4 red onion, thinly sliced
- 1/4 cup chopped fresh parsley
- 2 tablespoons olive oil
- 1 tablespoon lemon juice
- 1 clove garlic, minced
- Salt and pepper to taste
- Optional: crumbled feta cheese, sliced olives, chopped fresh basil

Instructions:

1. In a large mixing bowl, combine chickpeas, diced cucumber, halved cherry tomatoes, thinly sliced red onion, and chopped fresh parsley.

2. In a small bowl, whisk together olive oil, lemon juice, minced garlic, salt, and pepper to make the dressing.

3. Pour the dressing over the chickpea salad and toss gently to coat all the ingredients evenly.

4. Taste the salad and adjust seasoning if needed, adding more salt, pepper, or lemon juice as desired.

5. If using, sprinkle crumbled feta cheese, sliced olives, or chopped fresh basil over the top of the salad.

6. Serve the chickpea salad immediately, or cover and refrigerate for at least 30 minutes to allow the flavors to meld together before serving.

This chickpea salad with cucumbers and tomatoes is a light and refreshing dish that's perfect for picnics, potlucks, or as a healthy side dish for any meal. Enjoy its vibrant flavors and satisfying textures!

52. Quinoa and black bean enchiladas

Ingredients:
- 1 cup quinoa, rinsed
- 2 cups vegetable broth or water
- 1 can (15 oz) black beans,
drained and rinsed
- 1 cup corn kernels (fresh,
canned, or thawed if frozen)
- 1 red bell pepper, diced
- 1/2 red onion, diced
- 2 cloves garlic, minced
- 1 teaspoon ground cumin
- 1 teaspoon chili powder
- Salt and pepper to taste
- 8 large flour tortillas
- 2 cups enchilada sauce
- 1 cup shredded cheese (cheddar,
Monterey Jack, or Mexican blend)
- Chopped fresh cilantro for garnish
(optional)
- Sour cream, avocado, or salsa for serving
(optional)

Instructions:
1. Preheat your oven to 375°F (190°C). Grease a 9x13 inch baking dish.

2. In a saucepan, combine quinoa and vegetable broth or water. Bring to a boil, then reduce heat, cover, and simmer for about 15-20 minutes, or until quinoa is cooked and liquid is absorbed. Remove from heat and let it cool.

3. In a large mixing bowl, combine cooked quinoa, black beans, corn kernels, diced red bell pepper, diced red onion, minced garlic, ground cumin, chili powder, salt, and pepper. Mix until well combined.

4. Warm the flour tortillas in the microwave or in a skillet for a few seconds to make them pliable.

5. Spoon a generous amount of the quinoa and black bean mixture onto each tortilla, then roll it up tightly to enclose the filling. Place the rolled enchiladas seam-side down in the prepared baking dish.

6. Pour enchilada sauce evenly over the top of the rolled enchiladas, making sure they are all coated.

7. Sprinkle shredded cheese over the top of the enchiladas.

8. Cover the baking dish with foil and bake in the preheated oven for 20-25 minutes, or until the enchiladas are heated through and the cheese is melted and bubbly.

9. Remove from the oven and garnish with chopped fresh cilantro, if using. Serve the quinoa and black bean enchiladas hot, with sour cream, avocado, or salsa on the side if desired.

53. Greek yogurt with pineapple and coconut flakes

Ingredients:
- 1 cup Greek yogurt
- 1/2 cup diced pineapple (fresh or canned)
- 2 tablespoons unsweetened coconut flakes

Instructions:

1. Spoon Greek yogurt into a serving bowl or dish.

2. Top the Greek yogurt with diced pineapple.

3. Sprinkle unsweetened coconut flakes over the pineapple.

4. Serve immediately and enjoy this refreshing Greek yogurt with pineapple and coconut flakes!

This combination of creamy Greek yogurt, sweet pineapple, and crunchy coconut flakes will transport you to a tropical paradise with every bite. It's perfect for a quick and nutritious breakfast, snack, or dessert!

54. Tofu scramble breakfast burrito

Ingredients:
- 1 block (14 oz) firm tofu, drained and crumbled
- 1 tablespoon olive oil
- 1/2 onion, diced
- 1 bell pepper, diced
- 2 cloves garlic, minced
- 1 teaspoon ground cumin
- 1/2 teaspoon turmeric
- Salt and pepper to taste
- 4 large flour tortillas
- 1 cup cooked black beans
- 1 avocado, sliced
- Salsa, hot sauce, or chopped fresh cilantro for serving (optional)

Instructions:
1. Heat olive oil in a large skillet over medium heat. Add diced onion and bell pepper, and cook until softened, about 5 minutes.

2. Add minced garlic to the skillet and cook for another minute until fragrant.

3. Add crumbled tofu to the skillet, along with ground cumin, turmeric, salt, and pepper. Stir well to combine.

4. Cook the tofu mixture for 5-7 minutes, stirring occasionally, until heated through and slightly browned.

5. Warm the flour tortillas in a dry skillet or microwave for a few seconds to make them pliable.

6. Spoon a portion of the tofu scramble onto each tortilla, then top with cooked black beans and sliced avocado.

7. If desired, add salsa, hot sauce, or chopped fresh cilantro on top of the filling.

8. Roll up the tortillas to form burritos, folding in the sides as you go.

9. Serve the tofu scramble breakfast burritos immediately, or wrap them in foil to keep warm until ready to eat.

Enjoy these flavorful tofu scramble breakfast burritos as a satisfying and nutritious way to start your day! They're packed with protein, fiber, and all the delicious flavors of a classic breakfast scramble.

55. Lentil and quinoa stuffed bell peppers

Ingredients:
- 4 large bell peppers, any color
- 1/2 cup dry quinoa, rinsed
- 1 cup vegetable broth or water
- 1 can (15 oz) lentils, drained and rinsed
- 1 small onion, finely chopped
- 2 cloves garlic, minced
- 1 cup diced tomatoes (fresh or canned)
- 1 teaspoon ground cumin
- 1 teaspoon paprika
- 1/2 teaspoon dried oregano
- Salt and pepper to taste
- 1 cup shredded cheese (cheddar, Monterey Jack, or vegan cheese)
- Chopped fresh parsley or cilantro for garnish (optional)
- Sour cream, salsa, or avocado for serving (optional)

Instructions:

1. Preheat your oven to 375°F (190°C). Grease a baking dish large enough to fit the bell peppers.

2. Cut the tops off the bell peppers and remove the seeds and membranes. Arrange the peppers upright in the prepared baking dish.

3. In a saucepan, combine quinoa and vegetable broth or water. Bring to a boil, then reduce heat, cover, and simmer for about 15 minutes, or until quinoa is cooked and liquid is absorbed. Remove from heat and let it cool.

4. In a large skillet, heat a little oil over medium heat. Add chopped onion and minced garlic, and cook until softened, about 3-4 minutes.

5. Add diced tomatoes, cooked quinoa, lentils, ground cumin, paprika, dried oregano, salt, and pepper to the skillet. Cook for another 3-4 minutes until heated through and well combined.

6. Spoon the quinoa and lentil mixture evenly into the hollowed-out bell peppers, pressing down gently to pack the filling.

7. Sprinkle shredded cheese over the top of each stuffed pepper. Cover the baking dish with foil and bake in the preheated oven for 25-30 minutes, or until the peppers are tender and the cheese is melted and bubbly.

8. Remove from the oven and garnish with chopped fresh parsley or cilantro, if using. Serve the lentil and quinoa stuffed bell peppers hot, with sour cream, salsa, or avocado on the side if desired.

Enjoy these flavorful and nutritious lentil and quinoa stuffed bell peppers as a satisfying vegetarian meal! They're packed with protein, fiber, and delicious flavors that everyone will love.

56. Tempeh and vegetable stir-fry with ginger sauce

Ingredients:
- 8 oz tempeh, cubed
- 2 tablespoons soy sauce or tamari
- 1 tablespoon sesame oil
- 1 tablespoon vegetable oil
- 2 cloves garlic, minced
- 1 tablespoon grated ginger
- 1 bell pepper, thinly sliced
- 1 carrot, julienned
- 1 cup broccoli florets
- 1/2 cup snow peas, trimmed
- 2 green onions, chopped
- Cooked rice or noodles for serving

For the Ginger Sauce:
- 1/4 cup soy sauce or tamari
- 2 tablespoons rice vinegar
- 1 tablespoon maple syrup or honey
- 1 tablespoon cornstarch
- 1 tablespoon grated ginger
- 1 clove garlic, minced
- 1/4 cup water

Instructions:
1. In a bowl, marinate cubed tempeh in soy sauce or tamari and sesame oil for 15-20 minutes.

2. In a small bowl, whisk together all ingredients for the ginger sauce until smooth. Set aside.

3. Heat vegetable oil in a large skillet or wok over medium-high heat. Add marinated tempeh and cook until browned and crispy, about 5-7 minutes. Remove tempeh from the skillet and set aside.

4. In the same skillet, add minced garlic and grated ginger. Stir-fry for 1 minute until fragrant.

5. Add thinly sliced bell pepper, julienned carrot, broccoli florets, and snow peas to the skillet. Stir-fry for 4-5 minutes until vegetables are tender-crisp.

6. Return cooked tempeh to the skillet, along with chopped green onions.

7. Give the ginger sauce a quick stir and then pour it into the skillet. Cook, stirring constantly, until the sauce thickens and coats the tempeh and vegetables, about 2-3 minutes.

8. Remove from heat and serve the tempeh and vegetable stir-fry hot, over cooked rice or noodles.

57. Protein-packed overnight oats with chia seeds and fruit

Ingredients:
- 1/2 cup rolled oats
- 1 tablespoon chia seeds
- 1/2 cup Greek yogurt
- 1/2 cup milk (dairy or plant-based)
- 1 tablespoon honey or maple syrup (optional)
- 1/2 teaspoon vanilla extract
- 1/2 cup diced fruit (such as berries, banana, or mango)
- 1 tablespoon nut butter (such as almond or peanut butter)
- Optional toppings: sliced almonds, shredded coconut, additional fruit

Instructions:

1. In a jar or container with a lid, combine rolled oats, chia seeds, Greek yogurt, milk, honey or maple syrup (if using), and vanilla extract. Stir well to combine all ingredients.

2. Gently fold in diced fruit and nut butter into the oat mixture.

3. Cover the jar or container with a lid and refrigerate overnight, or for at least 4 hours, to allow the oats and chia seeds to soak and soften.

4. When ready to serve, give the overnight oats a good stir. If the consistency is too thick, you can add a splash of milk to loosen it up.

5. Transfer the overnight oats to a bowl or enjoy directly from the jar.

6. Top with sliced almonds, shredded coconut, or additional fruit if desired.

Enjoy these protein-packed overnight oats with chia seeds and fruit as a delicious and satisfying breakfast option! They're easy to prepare ahead of time and can be customized with your favorite fruits and toppings for endless variety.

58. Black bean and avocado wrap with salsa

Ingredients:
- 1 large flour tortilla or wrap
- 1/2 cup canned black beans, drained and rinsed
- 1/2 avocado, sliced
- 2 tablespoons salsa
- Handful of shredded lettuce or spinach
- Optional: shredded cheese, sour cream, chopped cilantro

Instructions:
1. Warm the flour tortilla or wrap in a dry skillet or microwave for a few seconds to make it pliable.

2. Lay the tortilla flat on a clean surface.

3. Spread black beans evenly over the center of the tortilla.

4. Arrange sliced avocado on top of the black beans.

5. Spoon salsa over the avocado.

6. Add shredded lettuce or spinach on top of the salsa.

7. If desired, sprinkle shredded cheese, dollop sour cream, or sprinkle chopped cilantro over the filling.

8. Fold in the sides of the tortilla, then roll it up tightly from the bottom to enclose the filling.

9. Slice the wrap in half diagonally, if desired, and serve immediately.

Enjoy this flavorful and satisfying black bean and avocado wrap with salsa as a quick and easy lunch or dinner option! It's packed with protein, healthy fats, and fresh flavors.

59. Chickpea and vegetable stew

Ingredients:
- 1 tablespoon olive oil
- 1 onion, diced
- 2 cloves garlic, minced
- 2 carrots, diced
- 2 celery stalks, diced
- 1 bell pepper, diced
- 1 can (15 oz) chickpeas, drained and rinsed
- 1 can (14 oz) diced tomatoes
- 4 cups vegetable broth
- 1 teaspoon dried thyme
- 1 teaspoon dried rosemary
- Salt and pepper to taste
- Chopped fresh parsley for garnish (optional)

Instructions:

1. Heat olive oil in a large pot or Dutch oven over medium heat.

2. Add diced onion and minced garlic to the pot. Cook, stirring occasionally, until softened and fragrant, about 5 minutes.

3. Add diced carrots, celery, and bell pepper to the pot. Cook for another 5 minutes until vegetables are slightly softened.

4. Stir in chickpeas, diced tomatoes (with their juices), vegetable broth, dried thyme, and dried rosemary. Season with salt and pepper to taste.

5. Bring the stew to a boil, then reduce heat to low, cover, and simmer for 20-25 minutes, or until vegetables are tender and flavors are well blended.

6. Taste and adjust seasoning if needed, adding more salt and pepper as desired.

7. Serve the chickpea and vegetable stew hot, garnished with chopped fresh parsley if desired.

Enjoy this hearty and nutritious chickpea and vegetable stew as a comforting meal on a chilly day! It's packed with fiber, protein, and vitamins from the chickpeas and vegetables, and it's sure to warm you up from the inside out.

60. Quinoa and vegetable sushi rolls

Ingredients:
- 1 cup sushi rice
- 2 cups water
- 2 tablespoons rice vinegar
- 1 tablespoon sugar
- 1/2 teaspoon salt
- 4 nori seaweed sheets
- 1 cup cooked quinoa
- 1/2 cucumber, julienned
- 1 carrot, julienned
- 1/2 avocado, sliced
- 4-6 asparagus spears, blanched and sliced lengthwise
- Soy sauce, pickled ginger, and wasabi for serving

Instructions:
1. Rinse sushi rice under cold water until the water runs clear. In a saucepan, combine sushi rice and water. Bring to a boil, then reduce heat to low, cover, and simmer for 15-20 minutes, or until rice is cooked and water is absorbed.

2. In a small bowl, mix rice vinegar, sugar, and salt until sugar and salt are dissolved. Gently fold the vinegar mixture into the cooked sushi rice. Let it cool to room temperature.

3. Place a bamboo sushi rolling mat on a clean surface, with the slats running horizontally. Lay a nori seaweed sheet shiny side down on the mat.

4. With wet hands, spread a thin layer of quinoa over the nori sheet, leaving a 1-inch border at the top edge.

5. Arrange cucumber, carrot, avocado, and asparagus slices in a single layer across the bottom edge of the nori sheet.

6. Using the bamboo mat, carefully roll up the nori sheet, tucking in the filling tightly as you go. Use a little water to seal the edge of the nori sheet.

7. Repeat with the remaining nori sheets and filling ingredients. Using a sharp knife dipped in water, slice each sushi roll into 6-8 pieces. Serve the quinoa and vegetable sushi rolls with soy sauce, pickled ginger, and wasabi for dipping.

Enjoy these homemade quinoa and vegetable sushi rolls as a nutritious and satisfying meal or snack! They're perfect for a light lunch or dinner and can be customized with your favorite vegetables and toppings.

61. Greek yogurt with mango and pistachios

Ingredients:
- 1 cup Greek yogurt
- 1 ripe mango, diced
- 2 tablespoons chopped pistachios

Instructions:

1. Spoon Greek yogurt into a serving bowl or dish.

2. Top the Greek yogurt with diced mango.

3. Sprinkle chopped pistachios over the mango.

4. Serve immediately and enjoy this refreshing Greek yogurt with mango and pistachios!

This combination of creamy Greek yogurt, sweet mango, and crunchy pistachios makes for a delightful and satisfying breakfast, snack, or dessert. Feel free to customize it with additional toppings such as honey or shredded coconut if desired!

62. Tofu and broccoli quiche with whole wheat crust

Ingredients:
- *Crust:*
  - 1 cup whole wheat flour
  - 1/4 teaspoon salt
  - 1/4 cup cold unsalted butter
  - 2-3 tablespoons cold water

- *Filling:*
  - 1 block (14 oz) firm tofu, crumbled
  - 1 tablespoon olive oil
  - 1 onion, diced
  - 2 cloves garlic, minced
  - 2 cups broccoli florets, blanched and chopped
  - 1/2 cup shredded cheese
  - 4 eggs (or substitute with tofu)
  - 1/2 cup milk

Instructions:

1. **Crust:** Mix flour, salt, and butter. Add water until dough forms. Chill, roll, and line a pie dish. Pre-bake for 10-12 minutes at 375°F (190°C).

2. **Filling:** Sauté onion and garlic. Add crumbled tofu, broccoli, cheese, and seasoning. In a separate bowl, whisk eggs (or tofu) and milk. Pour over tofu and broccoli mixture. Cook until set.

3. Pour filling into pre-baked crust. Bake for 25-30 minutes until set.

4. Serve and enjoy this nutritious quiche!

This version maintains the essential steps and ingredients for a delicious tofu and broccoli quiche with whole wheat crust, making it easier to follow while retaining the flavors and textures you love.

63. Lentil and vegetable curry with naan bread

Ingredients:
- 1 cup dried lentils
- 2 cups vegetable broth
- 1 tablespoon olive oil
- 1 onion, diced
- 2 cloves garlic, minced
- 1 tablespoon curry powder
- 1 teaspoon ground cumin
- 1 teaspoon ground coriander
- 1/2 teaspoon turmeric
- 1 can (14 oz) diced tomatoes
- 2 cups mixed vegetables (such as bell pepper, carrot, and cauliflower), chopped
- Salt and pepper to taste
- Naan bread, for serving

Instructions:
1. Rinse the lentils under cold water and drain. In a saucepan, combine lentils and vegetable broth. Bring to a boil, then reduce heat, cover, and simmer for 20-25 minutes, or until lentils are tender.

2. In a large skillet, heat olive oil over medium heat. Add diced onion and minced garlic, and cook until softened, about 5 minutes.

3. Add curry powder, ground cumin, ground coriander, and turmeric to the skillet. Cook for another minute until fragrant.

4. Stir in diced tomatoes (with their juices) and mixed vegetables. Cook for 5-7 minutes until vegetables are tender.

5. Add cooked lentils (and any remaining broth) to the skillet. Stir well to combine.

6. Season with salt and pepper to taste. Cook for another 2-3 minutes to heat through.

7. Serve the lentil and vegetable curry hot, with naan bread on the side.

Enjoy this flavorful and comforting lentil and vegetable curry with naan bread for a satisfying vegetarian meal! It's packed with protein, fiber, and aromatic spices that make it a delicious and nutritious dish.

64. Tempeh and avocado sandwich with whole grain bread

Ingredients:
- 8 oz tempeh, sliced
- 1 tablespoon olive oil
- 1 tablespoon soy sauce or tamari
- 4 slices whole grain bread
- 1 ripe avocado, sliced
- Lettuce leaves
- Tomato slices
- Mustard or mayonnaise (optional)
- Salt and pepper to taste

Instructions:

1. In a skillet, heat olive oil over medium heat. Add sliced tempeh and soy sauce (or tamari). Cook for 3-4 minutes on each side, or until golden brown and heated through. Remove from heat and set aside.

2. Toast whole grain bread slices until golden and crisp.

3. Spread mustard or mayonnaise (if using) on one side of each toasted bread slice.

4. Layer tempeh slices, avocado slices, lettuce leaves, and tomato slices on top of two bread slices.

5. Season with salt and pepper to taste.

6. Top with the remaining bread slices to form sandwiches. Slice in half if desired, and serve immediately.

Enjoy this delicious and nutritious tempeh and avocado sandwich with whole grain bread for a satisfying lunch or dinner option! It's packed with protein, healthy fats, and wholesome ingredients that will keep you feeling satisfied and energized.

65. Protein smoothie bowl with mixed berries and nuts

Ingredients:
- 1 ripe banana, frozen
- 1/2 cup mixed berries (such as strawberries, blueberries, raspberries)
- 1/2 cup Greek yogurt or plant-based yogurt
- 1 scoop protein powder (vanilla or berry-flavored)
- 1/4 cup milk (dairy or plant-based)
- Toppings: mixed nuts (such as almonds, walnuts, or pecans), fresh berries, shredded coconut, chia seeds

Instructions:

1. In a blender, combine frozen banana, mixed berries, Greek yogurt, protein powder, and milk.

2. Blend until smooth and creamy, adding more milk if needed to reach desired consistency.

3. Pour the smoothie into a bowl.

4. Top with mixed nuts, fresh berries, shredded coconut, and chia seeds.

5. Serve immediately and enjoy this protein-packed smoothie bowl for breakfast or as a satisfying snack!

This protein smoothie bowl with mixed berries and nuts is not only delicious but also nutritious, providing a balanced combination of protein, healthy fats, and fiber to keep you feeling full and energized throughout the day. Feel free to customize it with your favorite toppings!

66. Black bean and corn chowder

Ingredients:
- 1 tablespoon olive oil
- 1 onion, diced
- 2 cloves garlic, minced
- 2 carrots, diced
- 2 celery stalks, diced
- 1 bell pepper, diced
- 1 can (15 oz) black beans, drained and rinsed
- 1 can (15 oz) corn kernels, drained
- 4 cups vegetable broth
- 1 teaspoon ground cumin
- 1 teaspoon smoked paprika
- Salt and pepper to taste
- 1/2 cup heavy cream or coconut cream (optional)
- Fresh cilantro or green onions for garnish (optional)

Instructions:
1. In a large pot or Dutch oven, heat olive oil over medium heat. Add diced onion and minced garlic, and cook until softened, about 5 minutes.

2. Add diced carrots, celery, and bell pepper to the pot. Cook for another 5 minutes until vegetables are slightly softened.

3. Stir in drained black beans, drained corn kernels, vegetable broth, ground cumin, and smoked paprika. Season with salt and pepper to taste.

4. Bring the chowder to a boil, then reduce heat to low, cover, and simmer for 15-20 minutes, or until vegetables are tender and flavors are well blended.

5. If using, stir in heavy cream or coconut cream to add creaminess to the chowder. Cook for another 2-3 minutes until heated through.

6. Taste and adjust seasoning if needed.

7. Serve the black bean and corn chowder hot, garnished with fresh cilantro or green onions if desired.

Enjoy this hearty and comforting black bean and corn chowder as a satisfying meal on a chilly day! It's packed with protein, fiber, and delicious flavors that everyone will love.

67. Chickpea and vegetable stir-fry with coconut milk

Ingredients:
- 1 can (15 oz) chickpeas, drained and rinsed
- 2 cups mixed vegetables (such as bell peppers, broccoli, snap peas, carrots), chopped
- 1 onion, thinly sliced
- 3 cloves garlic, minced
- 1-inch piece of ginger, minced
- 1 can (14 oz) coconut milk
- 2 tablespoons soy sauce (or tamari for gluten-free)
- 1 tablespoon curry powder
- 1 tablespoon vegetable oil
- Salt and pepper to taste
- Cooked rice or noodles for serving
- Chopped fresh cilantro or green onions for garnish (optional)

Instructions:
1. Heat vegetable oil in a large skillet or wok over medium-high heat.

2. Add sliced onion and cook until translucent, about 2-3 minutes.

3. Add minced garlic and ginger, cook for another minute until fragrant.

4. Add chopped mixed vegetables to the skillet. Stir-fry for 3-4 minutes until they start to soften but still retain their crunch.

5. Stir in chickpeas and continue cooking for another 2 minutes.

6. In a small bowl, whisk together coconut milk, soy sauce, and curry powder until well combined.

7. Pour the coconut milk mixture into the skillet with the vegetables and chickpeas. Stir well to combine.

8. Bring the mixture to a simmer and let it cook for 5-7 minutes, allowing the flavors to meld and the sauce to thicken slightly.

9. Season with salt and pepper to taste. Serve the stir-fry hot over cooked rice or noodles. Garnish with chopped cilantro or green onions if desired.

68. Quinoa salad with roasted vegetables and feta

Ingredients:
- 1 cup quinoa, rinsed
- 2 cups water or vegetable broth
- 2 cups mixed vegetables (such as bell peppers, zucchini, cherry tomatoes, red onion), chopped
- 2 tablespoons olive oil
- Salt and pepper to taste
- 1/2 cup crumbled feta cheese
- 1/4 cup chopped fresh parsley or basil
- 2 tablespoons lemon juice
- 2 tablespoons balsamic vinegar
- Optional: 1/4 cup toasted pine nuts or almonds

Instructions:
1. Preheat your oven to 400°F (200°C).

2. In a saucepan, combine quinoa and water or vegetable broth. Bring to a boil, then reduce heat to low, cover, and simmer for 15-20 minutes, or until quinoa is cooked and water is absorbed. Remove from heat and let it sit, covered, for 5 minutes. Fluff with a fork and set aside to cool.

3. While the quinoa is cooking, spread the chopped mixed vegetables on a baking sheet. Drizzle with olive oil and season with salt and pepper. Toss to coat evenly.

4. Roast the vegetables in the preheated oven for 20-25 minutes, or until they are tender and slightly caramelized, stirring halfway through.

5. In a large bowl, combine the cooked quinoa, roasted vegetables, crumbled feta cheese, and chopped parsley or basil.

6. In a small bowl, whisk together lemon juice and balsamic vinegar. Pour the dressing over the salad and toss to combine.

7. Taste and adjust seasoning if needed.

8. If using, sprinkle toasted pine nuts or almonds over the salad before serving. Serve the quinoa salad at room temperature or chilled.

69. Greek yogurt with figs and walnuts

Ingredients:
- 1 cup Greek yogurt
- 2-3 fresh figs, sliced
- 2 tablespoons chopped walnuts
- 1 tablespoon honey (optional, for drizzling)
- Pinch of cinnamon (optional)

Instructions:
1. Spoon the Greek yogurt into a serving bowl or individual serving dishes.

2. Arrange the sliced figs on top of the yogurt.

3. Sprinkle chopped walnuts over the figs and yogurt.

4. If desired, drizzle honey over the yogurt and toppings.

5. Optionally, sprinkle a pinch of cinnamon over the top for extra flavor.

6. Serve immediately and enjoy!

This Greek Yogurt with Figs and Walnuts makes for a nutritious and satisfying breakfast or snack option. Feel free to adjust the toppings and sweetness according to your taste preferences.

70. Tofu and vegetable pad thai

Ingredients:
- 8 oz (225g) rice noodles
- 1 block (14 oz) extra-firm tofu, pressed and cubed
- 2 tablespoons vegetable oil
- 2 cloves garlic, minced
- 1 tablespoon rice vinegar
- 1 teaspoon Sriracha sauce (adjust to taste)
- Salt to taste
- Chopped peanuts, lime wedges, and fresh cilantro for serving
- 1 small onion, thinly sliced
- 2 cups mixed vegetables (such as bell peppers, bean sprouts, carrots, broccoli), thinly sliced or julienned
- 2 eggs, beaten (optional)
- 3 tablespoons soy sauce
- 2 tablespoons tamarind paste
- 2 tablespoons brown sugar (adjust to taste)

Instructions:
1. Cook the rice noodles according to the package instructions until al dente. Drain and set aside.

2. In a small bowl, mix together soy sauce, tamarind paste, brown sugar, rice vinegar, and Sriracha sauce to make the sauce. Set aside.

3. Heat 1 tablespoon of vegetable oil in a large skillet or wok over medium-high heat. Add the cubed tofu and cook until golden brown on all sides. Remove the tofu from the skillet and set aside.

4. In the same skillet, add another tablespoon of vegetable oil. Add minced garlic and sliced onion, and sauté until fragrant and translucent.

5. If using eggs, push the vegetables to one side of the skillet and pour the beaten eggs into the empty space. Scramble the eggs until cooked through, then mix with the vegetables.

6. Add the mixed vegetables to the skillet and stir-fry for 3-4 minutes until they start to soften but still retain their crunch.

7. Add the cooked rice noodles and tofu back to the skillet.

8. Pour the prepared sauce over the noodles and tofu. Toss everything together until well combined and heated through. Taste and adjust seasoning with salt or more soy sauce if needed.

9. Serve the tofu and vegetable pad thai hot, garnished with chopped peanuts, lime wedges, and fresh cilantro.

71. Lentil and sweet potato shepherd's pie

Ingredients:
***Filling*:**
- 1 cup dry lentils
- 2 cups vegetable broth
- 1 tbsp olive oil
- 1 onion, diced
- 2 cloves garlic, minced
- 2 carrots, diced
- 2 stalks celery, diced
- 1 bell pepper, diced
- 1 cup frozen peas
- 2 tbsp tomato paste
- 1 tbsp soy sauce
- 1 tsp dried thyme
- Salt and pepper

Topping:
- 2 large sweet potatoes, peeled and cubed
- 2 tbsp butter or olive oil
- 1/4 cup milk
- Salt and pepper

Instructions:
1. Cook lentils in broth until tender, then drain.

2. Sauté onion, garlic, carrots, celery, and bell pepper in olive oil until soft.

3. Add cooked lentils, peas, tomato paste, soy sauce, thyme, salt, and pepper to the skillet.

4. Mash boiled sweet potatoes with butter, milk, salt, and pepper.

5. Spread lentil mixture in a baking dish, top with mashed sweet potatoes.

6. Bake at 375°F (190°C) for 25-30 minutes until golden and bubbly.

7. Let cool slightly before serving.

Enjoy your Lentil and Sweet Potato Shepherd's Pie!

72. Tempeh bacon and avocado Caesar salad

Ingredients:
For the Tempeh Bacon:
- 1 block (8 oz) tempeh, thinly sliced
- 2 tablespoons soy sauce or tamari
- 1 tablespoon maple syrup
- 1 tablespoon apple cider vinegar
- 1 teaspoon smoked paprika
- 1/2 teaspoon garlic powder
- 1 tablespoon olive oil (for frying)

For the Salad:
- 1 head romaine lettuce, chopped
- 1 ripe avocado, sliced
- 1/4 cup vegan Caesar dressing (store-bought or homemade)
- 2 tablespoons nutritional yeast (optional, for extra flavor)
- Salt and pepper to taste

Instructions:
For the Tempeh Bacon:
1. In a shallow dish, whisk together soy sauce, maple syrup, apple cider vinegar, smoked paprika, and garlic powder.

2. Add the thinly sliced tempeh to the marinade, ensuring each slice is well coated. Let it marinate for at least 15 minutes.

3. Heat olive oil in a skillet over medium heat. Add the marinated tempeh slices and cook for 3-4 minutes on each side, or until crispy and browned. Remove from heat and set aside.

For the Salad:
1. In a large salad bowl, combine chopped romaine lettuce and sliced avocado.

2. Drizzle vegan Caesar dressing over the salad and toss gently to coat the leaves evenly.

3. Sprinkle nutritional yeast over the salad for extra flavor, if desired.

4. Season with salt and pepper to taste.

5. Top the salad with the cooked tempeh bacon slices.

6. Serve immediately and enjoy your Tempeh Bacon and Avocado Caesar Salad!

73. Protein-packed banana bread with walnuts

Ingredients:
- 1 1/2 cups mashed ripe bananas (about 3 large bananas)
- 1/3 cup Greek yogurt
- 1/4 cup honey or maple syrup
- 1/4 cup milk (dairy or non-dairy)
- 2 eggs
- 1 teaspoon vanilla extract
- 1 3/4 cups whole wheat flour or all-purpose flour
- 1/4 cup vanilla protein powder
- 1 teaspoon baking powder
- 1/2 teaspoon baking soda
- 1/2 teaspoon salt
- 1/2 cup chopped walnuts (plus extra for topping, if desired)

Instructions:

1. Preheat your oven to 350°F (175°C). Grease or line a 9x5-inch loaf pan with parchment paper.

2. In a large mixing bowl, combine the mashed bananas, Greek yogurt, honey or maple syrup, milk, eggs, and vanilla extract. Mix until well combined.

3. In a separate bowl, whisk together the whole wheat flour (or all-purpose flour), protein powder, baking powder, baking soda, and salt.

4. Gradually add the dry ingredients to the wet ingredients, stirring until just combined. Be careful not to overmix.

5. Gently fold in the chopped walnuts.

6. Pour the batter into the prepared loaf pan, spreading it out evenly.

7. If desired, sprinkle additional chopped walnuts over the top of the batter.

8. Bake in the preheated oven for 50-60 minutes, or until a toothpick inserted into the center comes out clean.

9. Remove the banana bread from the oven and allow it to cool in the pan for 10 minutes before transferring it to a wire rack to cool completely. Once cooled, slice and serve. Enjoy your protein-packed banana bread with walnuts!

74. Black bean and corn stuffed zucchini

Ingredients:
- 4 medium zucchinis
- 1 can (15 oz) black beans, drained and rinsed
- 1 cup corn kernels (fresh, canned, or frozen)
- 1 red bell pepper, diced
- 1 small onion, diced
- 2 cloves garlic, minced
- 1 teaspoon ground cumin
- 1 teaspoon chili powder
- 1/2 teaspoon smoked paprika
- Salt and pepper to taste
- 1 cup shredded cheese (such as cheddar or Monterey Jack), divided
- Chopped fresh cilantro or green onions for garnish (optional)

Instructions:
1. Preheat your oven to 375°F (190°C). Grease a baking dish large enough to hold the zucchinis.

2. Cut each zucchini in half lengthwise. Use a spoon to scoop out the seeds and create a hollow space in each zucchini half. Place the hollowed-out zucchinis in the prepared baking dish.

3. In a large skillet, heat olive oil over medium heat. Add diced onion and bell pepper, and sauté until softened, about 5 minutes.

4. Add minced garlic to the skillet and cook for an additional minute, until fragrant.

5. Stir in black beans, corn kernels, ground cumin, chili powder, smoked paprika, salt, and pepper. Cook for another 3-4 minutes, allowing the flavors to meld together.

6. Remove the skillet from heat and stir in 1/2 cup of shredded cheese until melted and well combined.

7. Spoon the black bean and corn mixture evenly into the hollowed-out zucchini halves, pressing gently to pack the filling.

8. Sprinkle the remaining 1/2 cup of shredded cheese over the top of the stuffed zucchinis.
9. Cover the baking dish with aluminum foil and bake in the preheated oven for 20-25 minutes, or until the zucchinis are tender.

10. Remove the foil and bake for an additional 5-10 minutes, or until the cheese is melted and bubbly. Garnish with chopped cilantro or green onions, if desired, before serving.

Enjoy your flavorful Black Bean and Corn Stuffed Zucchini as a nutritious and satisfying meal!

75. Chickpea and spinach stuffed peppers

Ingredients:
- 4 large bell peppers, any color
- 1 can (15 oz) chickpeas, drained and rinsed
- 2 cups fresh spinach, chopped
- 1 small onion, finely chopped
- 2 cloves garlic, minced
- 1 teaspoon ground cumin
- 1 teaspoon ground coriander
- 1/2 teaspoon paprika
- Salt and pepper to taste
- 1 cup cooked quinoa or rice
- 1/2 cup shredded cheese (optional)
- Fresh parsley or cilantro for garnish (optional)

Instructions:

1. Preheat your oven to 375°F (190°C). Grease a baking dish large enough to hold the peppers.

2. Cut the tops off the bell peppers and remove the seeds and membranes. Place the hollowed-out peppers in the prepared baking dish.

3. In a large skillet, heat olive oil over medium heat. Add chopped onion and cook until translucent, about 5 minutes.

4. Add minced garlic to the skillet and cook for an additional minute, until fragrant.

5. Stir in chickpeas, chopped spinach, ground cumin, ground coriander, paprika, salt, and pepper. Cook for another 3-4 minutes until the spinach is wilted and the flavors are combined.

6. Remove the skillet from heat and stir in cooked quinoa or rice until well combined.

7. Spoon the chickpea and spinach mixture evenly into the hollowed-out bell peppers, pressing gently to pack the filling.

8. If using, sprinkle shredded cheese over the top of the stuffed peppers. Cover the baking dish with aluminum foil and bake in the preheated oven for 25-30 minutes, or until the peppers are tender.

9. Remove the foil and bake for an additional 5-10 minutes, or until the cheese is melted and bubbly. Garnish with fresh parsley or cilantro before serving.

76. Quinoa and vegetable stuffed tomatoes

Ingredients:
- 6 large tomatoes
- 1 cup cooked quinoa
- 1 small onion, finely chopped
- 2 cloves garlic, minced
- 1 bell pepper, diced
- 1 zucchini, diced
- 1 carrot, grated
- 1 cup spinach, chopped
- 1/4 cup fresh parsley, chopped
- 1 teaspoon dried oregano
- Salt and pepper to taste
- 1/2 cup shredded cheese (optional)
- Olive oil for drizzling

Instructions:
1. Preheat your oven to 375°F (190°C). Grease a baking dish large enough to hold the tomatoes.

2. Cut the tops off the tomatoes and scoop out the seeds and pulp to create hollow shells. Reserve the pulp for later use.

3. In a large skillet, heat olive oil over medium heat. Add chopped onion and cook until translucent, about 5 minutes.

4. Add minced garlic to the skillet and cook for an additional minute, until fragrant.

5. Stir in diced bell pepper, zucchini, and grated carrot. Cook for 5-7 minutes, until the vegetables are tender.

6. Add chopped spinach, cooked quinoa, dried oregano, salt, and pepper to the skillet. Cook for another 2-3 minutes, until the spinach is wilted and the flavors are combined.

7. Remove the skillet from heat and stir in chopped parsley and reserved tomato pulp.

8. Spoon the quinoa and vegetable mixture evenly into the hollowed-out tomatoes, pressing gently to pack the filling.

9. If using, sprinkle shredded cheese over the top of the stuffed tomatoes.

10. Place the stuffed tomatoes in the prepared baking dish. Drizzle with a little olive oil.

11. Bake in the preheated oven for 25-30 minutes, or until the tomatoes are tender and the filling is heated through. Serve hot, garnished with additional chopped parsley if desired.

77. Greek yogurt with cherries and dark chocolate chips

Ingredients:

- 1 cup Greek yogurt
- 1/2 cup fresh cherries, pitted and halved
- 2 tablespoons dark chocolate chips
- Honey or maple syrup (optional, for sweetness)

Instructions:

1. Spoon the Greek yogurt into a serving bowl.

2. Add the halved cherries on top of the yogurt.

3. Sprinkle dark chocolate chips over the yogurt and cherries.

4. If desired, drizzle honey or maple syrup over the yogurt for added sweetness.

5. Gently mix the ingredients together, or leave them layered for presentation.

6. Serve immediately and enjoy your delicious Greek Yogurt with Cherries and Dark Chocolate Chips!

This snack is not only tasty but also provides a balance of protein from the Greek yogurt, fiber and antioxidants from the cherries, and a hint of indulgence from the dark chocolate chips.

78. Tofu and vegetable curry with coconut milk

Ingredients:
- 1 block (14 oz) extra-firm tofu, pressed and cubed
- 2 tablespoons vegetable oil
- 1 onion, chopped
- 2 cloves garlic, minced
- 1-inch piece of ginger, minced
- 2 tablespoons curry powder
- 1 teaspoon ground turmeric
- 1 teaspoon ground cumin
- 1 can (14 oz) coconut milk
- 2 cups mixed vegetables (such as bell peppers, carrots, broccoli, snap peas), chopped
- Salt and pepper to taste
- Cooked rice or naan bread for serving
- Fresh cilantro for garnish (optional)

Instructions:

1. Heat vegetable oil in a large skillet or pot over medium heat.

2. Add chopped onion and cook until translucent, about 5 minutes.

3. Add minced garlic and ginger to the skillet, cook for another minute until fragrant.

4. Stir in curry powder, ground turmeric, and ground cumin. Cook for 1-2 minutes to toast the spices.

5. Add cubed tofu to the skillet and cook for 5-7 minutes, until lightly browned on all sides.

6. Pour in the coconut milk and stir to combine. Bring the mixture to a simmer.

7. Add chopped mixed vegetables to the skillet and stir well.

8. Cover the skillet and let the curry simmer for 10-15 minutes, or until the vegetables are tender.

9. Season with salt and pepper to taste. Serve the tofu and vegetable curry hot over cooked rice or with naan bread. Garnish with fresh cilantro if desired.

Enjoy your flavorful Tofu and Vegetable Curry with Coconut Milk! Adjust the spice level by adding more or less curry powder and chili flakes according to your taste preferences.

79. Lentil and vegetable stew with barley

Ingredients:
- 1 cup dry lentils, rinsed
- 1/2 cup pearl barley
- 6 cups vegetable broth
- 2 tablespoons olive oil
- 1 onion, chopped
- 2 carrots, diced
- 2 stalks celery, diced
- 2 cloves garlic, minced
- 1 bell pepper, chopped
- 1 can (14 oz) diced tomatoes
- 2 teaspoons dried thyme
- 1 teaspoon dried rosemary
- Salt and pepper to taste
- Fresh parsley for garnish (optional)

Instructions:

1. In a large pot, heat olive oil over medium heat. Add chopped onion, carrots, celery, and bell pepper. Cook until vegetables are softened, about 5-7 minutes.

2. Add minced garlic to the pot and cook for another minute until fragrant.

3. Stir in dry lentils and pearl barley. Cook for a couple of minutes to toast the lentils and barley.

4. Pour in vegetable broth and diced tomatoes (with their juices) into the pot. Add dried thyme, dried rosemary, salt, and pepper. Stir to combine.

5. Bring the mixture to a boil, then reduce the heat to low. Cover and simmer for 30-40 minutes, or until the lentils and barley are tender.

6. Taste and adjust seasoning if needed. Serve the lentil and vegetable stew hot, garnished with fresh parsley if desired.

Enjoy your hearty Lentil and Vegetable Stew with Barley! It's a comforting and nutritious meal that's perfect for chilly days.

80. Tempeh and vegetable fajitas with guacamole

For the Fajitas:
- 1 package (8 oz) tempeh, thinly sliced
- 2 bell peppers, sliced
- 1 onion, sliced
- 1 zucchini, sliced
- 2 tbsp olive oil
- 2 cloves garlic, minced
- 1 tsp chili powder
- 1/2 tsp ground cumin
- 1/2 tsp smoked paprika
- Salt and pepper
- 8 small tortillas

For the Guacamole:
- 2 ripe avocados
- 1 small tomato, diced
- 1/4 cup onion, finely chopped
- 1/4 cup cilantro, chopped
- 1-2 tbsp lime juice
- Salt and pepper

Instructions:
1. Sauté tempeh in olive oil until golden brown, then set aside.

2. Cook bell peppers, onion, and zucchini until tender-crisp, adding garlic and spices.

3. Return tempeh to skillet, toss with vegetables.

4. Warm tortillas.

5. For guacamole, mash avocados and mix with tomato, onion, cilantro, lime juice, salt, and pepper.

6. Serve fajita mixture in warm tortillas with guacamole on the side.

Enjoy your delicious Tempeh and Vegetable Fajitas with Guacamole!

81. Protein-packed chocolate avocado pudding

Ingredients:
- 2 ripe avocados
- 1/4 cup cocoa powder
- 1/4 cup honey or maple syrup (adjust to taste)
- 1 teaspoon vanilla extract
- 1/4 cup milk (dairy or non-dairy)
- 1 scoop chocolate protein powder
- Optional toppings: sliced bananas, berries, chopped nuts, shredded coconut

Instructions:
1. Cut the avocados in half and remove the pits. Scoop out the flesh into a blender or food processor.

2. Add cocoa powder, honey or maple syrup, vanilla extract, milk, and chocolate protein powder to the blender or food processor.

3. Blend until smooth and creamy, scraping down the sides as needed to ensure everything is well combined.

4. Taste and adjust sweetness if needed by adding more honey or maple syrup.

5. Transfer the pudding to serving bowls or glasses.

6. Chill in the refrigerator for at least 30 minutes before serving to allow the pudding to set.

7. Serve chilled, topped with your favorite toppings such as sliced bananas, berries, chopped nuts, or shredded coconut.

Enjoy your delicious and nutritious Protein-Packed Chocolate Avocado Pudding as a satisfying dessert or snack!

82. Black bean and corn salad with avocado dressing

Ingredients:
For the Salad:
- 2 cups cooked black beans
(or 1 can, drained and rinsed)
- 1 cup corn kernels
 (fresh, canned, or thawed if frozen)
- 1 red bell pepper, diced
- 1/2 red onion, finely chopped
- 1/4 cup chopped fresh cilantro
- Juice of 1 lime
- Salt and pepper to taste
- Optional: diced avocado for garnish

For the Avocado Dressing:
- 1 ripe avocado
- 1/4 cup plain Greek yogurt
- 2 tablespoons lime juice
- 2 tablespoons olive oil
- 1 clove garlic, minced
- 1/4 teaspoon ground cumin
- Salt and pepper to taste
- Water, as needed to thin the dressing

Instructions:

1. In a large mixing bowl, combine the cooked black beans, corn kernels, diced bell pepper, finely chopped red onion, and chopped fresh cilantro.

2. Squeeze the juice of one lime over the salad ingredients and toss gently to combine.

3. Season the salad with salt and pepper to taste. Set aside while you prepare the avocado dressing.

4. In a blender or food processor, combine the flesh of one ripe avocado, plain Greek yogurt, lime juice, olive oil, minced garlic, ground cumin, salt, and pepper.

5. Blend until smooth and creamy. If the dressing is too thick, add water, 1 tablespoon at a time, until you reach your desired consistency.

6. Taste the dressing and adjust seasoning if needed.

7. Pour the avocado dressing over the salad and toss gently to coat the ingredients evenly.

8. Optional: Garnish the salad with diced avocado before serving.

9. Serve the black bean and corn salad immediately, or chill in the refrigerator for 30 minutes to allow the flavors to meld together before serving.

83. Chickpea and kale Caesar salad

Salad:
- 1 bunch kale, torn
- 1 can (15 oz) chickpeas, roasted
- 1/4 cup grated Parmesan cheese
- 1/4 cup toasted bread crumbs
- Optional: cherry tomatoes, cucumber, avocado

Dressing:
- 1/2 cup Greek yogurt
- 2 tbsp lemon juice
- 2 tbsp grated Parmesan cheese
- 1 tbsp Dijon mustard
- 1 clove garlic, minced
- 1 tsp Worcestershire sauce
- Salt and pepper
- 2-3 tbsp olive oil

Instructions:
1. Combine torn kale, roasted chickpeas, Parmesan, and bread crumbs in a bowl.

2. Optionally, add tomatoes, cucumber, and avocado.

3. Whisk together yogurt, lemon juice, Parmesan, mustard, garlic, Worcestershire, salt, pepper, and olive oil.

4. Drizzle dressing over salad and toss to coat.

5. Serve immediately or chill briefly.

Enjoy your quick and delicious Chickpea and Kale Caesar Salad!

84. Quinoa and vegetable stir-fry with soy sauce

Ingredients:
- 1 cup quinoa, rinsed
- 2 cups water or vegetable broth
- 2 tablespoons oil (vegetable, sesame, or olive oil)
- 2 cloves garlic, minced
- 1 onion, thinly sliced
- 2 carrots, julienned or thinly sliced
- 1 bell pepper, thinly sliced
- 1 cup broccoli florets
- 1 cup snap peas or snow peas
- 1/4 cup soy sauce
- 2 tablespoons rice vinegar or apple cider vinegar
- 1 tablespoon sesame oil (optional)
- Optional toppings: sliced green onions, sesame seeds, chopped cilantro

Instructions:
1. In a medium saucepan, combine the rinsed quinoa and water or vegetable broth. Bring to a boil, then reduce the heat to low. Cover and simmer for 15-20 minutes, or until the quinoa is cooked and the liquid is absorbed. Remove from heat and let it sit covered for 5 minutes. Fluff with a fork and set aside.

2. In a large skillet or wok, heat the oil over medium-high heat. Add the minced garlic and sliced onion, and sauté for 2-3 minutes until fragrant and translucent.

3. Add the julienned carrots, thinly sliced bell pepper, broccoli florets, and snap peas to the skillet. Stir-fry for 5-7 minutes, or until the vegetables are tender-crisp.

4. In a small bowl, whisk together the soy sauce, rice vinegar, and sesame oil (if using). Pour the sauce over the cooked vegetables in the skillet.

5. Add the cooked quinoa to the skillet with the vegetables and sauce. Stir well to combine and coat everything evenly with the sauce. Cook for an additional 2-3 minutes to heat through.

6. Remove from heat and taste, adjusting seasoning if needed. Serve the quinoa and vegetable stir-fry hot, garnished with sliced green onions, sesame seeds, and chopped cilantro if desired.

Enjoy your flavorful and nutritious Quinoa and Vegetable Stir-Fry with Soy Sauce! It's a satisfying and versatile dish that's perfect for a quick and healthy meal.

85. Greek yogurt with strawberries and honey

Ingredients:

- 1 cup Greek yogurt
- 1/2 cup fresh strawberries, sliced
- 1-2 tablespoons honey (adjust to taste)
- Optional toppings: chopped nuts, granola, or mint leaves

Instructions:

1. Spoon the Greek yogurt into a serving bowl or individual cups.

2. Arrange the sliced strawberries on top of the yogurt.

3. Drizzle honey over the yogurt and strawberries, adjusting the amount to your taste preference.

4. Optionally, sprinkle chopped nuts or granola over the top for added crunch and flavor.

5. Garnish with fresh mint leaves for a refreshing touch if desired.

6. Serve immediately and enjoy your delicious Greek Yogurt with Strawberries and Honey!

This simple and nutritious snack or breakfast is bursting with flavor and provides a perfect balance of creamy, tangy, and sweet elements.

86. Tofu and vegetable bibimbap

Ingredients:
For the Tofu Marinade:
- 1 block (14 oz) firm tofu,
drained and pressed
- 2 tablespoons soy sauce
- 1 tablespoon sesame oil
- 1 tablespoon honey or maple syrup
- 2 cloves garlic, minced
- 1 teaspoon grated ginger
- Optional: 1 tablespoon gochujang
(Korean chili paste) for extra flavor and spice

For the Bibimbap:
- Cooked rice (white or brown)
- 2 cups mixed vegetables (such as
carrots, spinach, mushrooms,
zucchini, bean sprouts)
- 2 tablespoons vegetable oil
- 4 eggs (optional)
- Sesame seeds, for garnish
- Sliced green onions, for garnish
- Kimchi, for serving (optional)
- Gochujang, for serving (optional)

Instructions:
For the Tofu:
1. In a shallow dish, whisk together soy sauce, sesame oil, honey or maple syrup, minced garlic, and grated ginger (and gochujang if using).

2. Cut the pressed tofu into cubes or slices and add them to the marinade, ensuring they are well coated. Let marinate for at least 30 minutes, or longer for more flavor.

For the Bibimbap:
1. Cook rice according to package instructions and set aside.
2. Heat vegetable oil in a large skillet or wok over medium-high heat.

3. Add the marinated tofu to the skillet and cook until browned and crispy on all sides, about 5-7 minutes. Remove from the skillet and set aside.

4. In the same skillet, stir-fry the mixed vegetables until tender-crisp, adding a little more oil if needed. Season with salt and pepper to taste.

5. If using, fry eggs sunny-side-up or over-easy in the skillet.

6. To assemble bibimbap bowls, divide the cooked rice among serving bowls. Arrange the cooked tofu and stir-fried vegetables on top of the rice.

7. Place a fried egg on top of each bowl, if using.

8. Garnish with sesame seeds and sliced green onions. Serve hot with kimchi and gochujang on the side, if desired.

87. Lentil and vegetable pot pie

Filling:
- 1 cup dry lentils, rinsed
- 3 cups vegetable broth
- 2 tbsp olive oil
- 1 onion, diced
- 2 carrots, diced
- 2 celery stalks, diced
- 2 cloves garlic, minced
- 1 tsp each dried thyme and rosemary
- 1/2 tsp smoked paprika
- Salt and pepper
- 1 cup each frozen peas and corn
- 1/4 cup flour
- 1 cup unsweetened almond milk

Pie Crust:
- 2 1/2 cups all-purpose flour
- 1 cup cold unsalted butter, cubed
- 1/2 tsp salt
- 6-8 tbsp ice water

Instructions:
1. Cook lentils in vegetable broth until tender. Drain and set aside.

2. Sauté onion, carrots, celery, garlic, spices. Add peas, corn, cooked lentils, and flour. Stir in almond milk until thickened.

3. For the crust, mix flour, salt, and cold butter until crumbly. Add ice water until dough forms. Chill.

4. Roll out dough, place in pie dish. Add filling. Top with second crust, seal edges, and vent.

5. Bake at 400°F (200°C) for 35-40 mins until golden and bubbly.

Enjoy your comforting Lentil and Vegetable Pot Pie!

88. Tempeh and vegetable kebabs with barbecue sauce

Ingredients:
For the Kebabs:
- 1 block (8 oz) tempeh, cut into cubes
- 1 bell pepper, cut into chunks
- 1 zucchini, sliced
- 1 red onion, cut into chunks
- 8-10 cherry tomatoes
- Wooden or metal skewers, soaked in water if wooden

For the Barbecue Sauce:
- 1/2 cup ketchup
- 2 tablespoons soy sauce
- 2 tablespoons maple syrup or honey
- 1 tablespoon apple cider vinegar
- 1 teaspoon smoked paprika
- 1/2 teaspoon garlic powder
- Salt and pepper to taste

Instructions:

1. If using wooden skewers, soak them in water for at least 30 minutes to prevent burning.

2. Preheat your grill or grill pan over medium-high heat.

3. Thread the tempeh cubes, bell pepper chunks, zucchini slices, red onion chunks, and cherry tomatoes onto the skewers, alternating between ingredients.

4. In a small bowl, whisk together the ingredients for the barbecue sauce until well combined.

5. Brush the barbecue sauce generously over the assembled kebabs, reserving some sauce for basting during grilling.

6. Place the kebabs on the preheated grill or grill pan and cook for 8-10 minutes, turning occasionally, until the vegetables are tender and slightly charred, and the tempeh is heated through.

7. During grilling, brush the kebabs with additional barbecue sauce for extra flavor.

8. Once cooked, remove the kebabs from the grill and let them cool slightly before serving.

9. Serve the Tempeh and Vegetable Kebabs with extra barbecue sauce on the side for dipping, if desired.

Enjoy your delicious Tempeh and Vegetable Kebabs with Barbecue Sauce! They make a fantastic vegetarian option for grilling and are perfect for summer gatherings or weeknight dinners.

89. Protein-packed banana walnut muffins

Ingredients:
- 1 cup whole wheat flour
- 1 cup oat flour (or blended oats)
- 1/2 cup protein powder (vanilla or unflavored)
- 1 teaspoon baking soda
- 1/2 teaspoon salt
- 3 ripe bananas, mashed
- 2 large eggs
- 1/2 cup Greek yogurt
- 1/4 cup honey or maple syrup
- 1/4 cup coconut oil, melted
- 1 teaspoon vanilla extract
- 1/2 cup chopped walnuts

Instructions:

1. Preheat oven to 350°F (175°C) and line a muffin tin with paper liners or lightly grease it.

2. In a large bowl, combine whole wheat flour, oat flour, protein powder, baking soda, and salt.

3. In another bowl, mix mashed bananas, eggs, Greek yogurt, honey or maple syrup, melted coconut oil, and vanilla extract until well combined.

4. Add the wet ingredients to the dry ingredients and mix until just combined.

5. Fold in the chopped walnuts.

6. Divide the batter evenly among the muffin cups.

7. Bake for 18-20 minutes, or until a toothpick inserted into the center comes out clean

8. Let the muffins cool in the tin for 5 minutes, then transfer to a wire rack to cool completely.

Enjoy your nutritious and delicious Protein-Packed Banana Walnut Muffins! They make a great snack or breakfast option.

90. Black bean and corn stuffed mushrooms

Ingredients:
- 12 large mushrooms, stems removed
- 1 can (15 oz) black beans, drained and rinsed
- 1 cup corn kernels (fresh, canned, or thawed if frozen)
- 1/2 cup red bell pepper, finely diced
- 1/4 cup red onion, finely diced
- 2 cloves garlic, minced
- 1 teaspoon ground cumin
- 1 teaspoon chili powder
- Salt and pepper to taste
- 1/4 cup shredded cheese (optional, for a vegan option use dairy-free cheese)
- 2 tablespoons olive oil
- Fresh cilantro, chopped (for garnish)

Instructions:
1. Preheat oven to 375°F (190°C) and line a baking sheet with parchment paper.

2. Heat olive oil in a skillet over medium heat. Add garlic, red onion, and bell pepper. Sauté for 3-4 minutes until softened.

3. Add black beans, corn, ground cumin, chili powder, salt, and pepper. Cook for another 2-3 minutes, stirring well. Remove from heat.

4. Arrange mushroom caps on the prepared baking sheet. Spoon the black bean and corn mixture into each mushroom cap.

5. Sprinkle shredded cheese on top of each stuffed mushroom if using.

6. Bake for 20-25 minutes, or until the mushrooms are tender and the cheese is melted and golden.

7. Remove from oven and let cool slightly. Garnish with fresh cilantro.

Enjoy your flavorful and nutritious Black Bean and Corn Stuffed Mushrooms! They make a great appetizer or side dish.

91. Chickpea and roasted vegetable pasta

Ingredients:
- 8 oz (225g) pasta (your choice)
- 1 can (15 oz) chickpeas, drained and rinsed
- 1 zucchini, diced
- 1 bell pepper, diced
- 1 red onion, diced
- 1 cup cherry tomatoes, halved
- 3 cloves garlic, minced
- 3 tablespoons olive oil
- 1 teaspoon dried oregano
- 1 teaspoon dried basil
- Salt and pepper to taste
- Fresh basil or parsley, chopped (for garnish)
- Optional: Grated Parmesan cheese or nutritional yeast for topping

Instructions:
1. Preheat oven to 400°F (200°C). Line a baking sheet with parchment paper.

2. In a large bowl, combine diced zucchini, bell pepper, red onion, cherry tomatoes, and chickpeas. Add minced garlic, olive oil, dried oregano, dried basil, salt, and pepper. Toss to coat evenly.

3. Spread the vegetable and chickpea mixture on the prepared baking sheet. Roast in the preheated oven for 20-25 minutes, or until the vegetables are tender and slightly charred.

4. While the vegetables are roasting, cook the pasta according to the package instructions. Drain and set aside.

5. Once the vegetables are done, combine them with the cooked pasta in a large bowl. Toss to mix well.

6. Garnish with fresh basil or parsley. Add grated Parmesan cheese or nutritional yeast if desired.

Enjoy your delicious Chickpea and Roasted Vegetable Pasta! It's a wholesome and satisfying meal perfect for any day of the week.

92. Quinoa and black bean salad with cilantro lime dressing

Ingredients
For the Cilantro Lime Dressing:
- 1/4 cup fresh lime juice
- 2 tablespoons olive oil
- 2 tablespoons fresh cilantro, chopped
- 1 clove garlic, minced
- 1 teaspoon honey or maple syrup
- Salt and pepper to taste

For the Salad:
- 1 cup quinoa, rinsed
- 1 can (15 oz) black beans, drained and rinsed
- 1 red bell pepper, diced
- 1 cup corn kernels (fresh, canned, or thawed if frozen)
- 1/4 cup red onion, finely chopped
- 1/4 cup fresh cilantro, chopped
- Salt and pepper to taste
- Optional toppings: avocado slices, cherry tomatoes, diced cucumber

Instructions:
1. In a medium saucepan, combine quinoa with 2 cups of water. Bring to a boil, then reduce heat to low, cover, and simmer for 15-20 minutes, or until quinoa is cooked and water is absorbed. Remove from heat and let it cool.

2. In a large bowl, combine cooked quinoa, black beans, diced red bell pepper, corn kernels, chopped red onion, and chopped cilantro. Season with salt and pepper to taste. Toss to combine.

3. In a small bowl, whisk together lime juice, olive oil, chopped cilantro, minced garlic, honey or maple syrup, salt, and pepper to make the cilantro lime dressing.

4. Pour the dressing over the quinoa and black bean salad and toss until everything is evenly coated.

5. Taste and adjust seasoning if needed.

6. Serve the quinoa and black bean salad chilled or at room temperature, garnished with additional cilantro leaves if desired.

7. Optional: Serve with avocado slices, cherry tomatoes, or diced cucumber on top for extra freshness and flavor.

**Enjoy your refreshing and nutritious Quinoa and Black Bean Salad with Cilantro Lime Dressing! It's perfect for a light lunch or as a side dish for any meal.**

93. Greek yogurt with raspberries and almonds

Ingredients:

- 1 cup Greek yogurt
- 1/2 cup fresh raspberries
- 2 tablespoons sliced almonds
- 1-2 teaspoons honey or maple syrup (optional)

Instructions:

1. Spoon the Greek yogurt into a serving bowl or individual cup.

2. Top with fresh raspberries and sliced almonds.

3. Drizzle with honey or maple syrup if desired.

4. Serve immediately.

Enjoy your delicious and healthy Greek Yogurt with Raspberries and Almonds! It's perfect for breakfast, a snack, or a light dessert.

94. Tofu and vegetable lettuce wraps with hoisin sauce

Filling:
- 1 block (14 oz) firm tofu, crumbled
- 2 tbsp soy sauce
- 1 tbsp sesame oil
- 1 tbsp olive oil
- 2 cloves garlic, minced
- 1 tsp grated ginger
- 1 cup mixed diced vegetables
- Salt and pepper to taste
- Iceberg or butter lettuce leaves

Hoisin Sauce:
- 3 tbsp hoisin sauce
- 1 tbsp soy sauce
- 1 tbsp rice vinegar
- 1 tsp sesame oil
- 1 tsp honey or maple syrup (optional)
- 1 tbsp water (to thin, if needed)

Optional Toppings:
- Sliced green onions
- Chopped cilantro
- Sliced almonds or peanuts
- Sesame seeds

Instructions:
1. Cook tofu with soy sauce, sesame oil, olive oil, garlic, and ginger until browned.

2. Add mixed vegetables, cook until tender-crisp.

3. Mix hoisin sauce ingredients, adjust consistency with water if needed.

4. Spoon tofu and vegetable mixture onto lettuce leaves, drizzle with hoisin sauce, and garnish with toppings.

5. Serve immediately.

Enjoy your Tofu and Vegetable Lettuce Wraps with Hoisin Sauce—a flavorful and healthy dish!

95. Lentil and vegetable lasagna

Ingredients:
Filling:
- 1 cup dry lentils, rinsed
- 3 cups vegetable broth
- 1 tbsp olive oil
- 1 onion, diced
- 2 cloves garlic, minced
- 1 carrot, diced
- 1 zucchini, diced
- 1 bell pepper, diced
- 1 can (15 oz) crushed tomatoes
- 2 tsp dried Italian herbs
- Salt and pepper to taste

Layers:
- 9 lasagna noodles (oven-ready or pre-cooked)
- 2 cups shredded mozzarella cheese
- 1 cup ricotta cheese
- 1/4 cup grated Parmesan cheese (optional)
- Fresh basil for garnish (optional)

Instructions:
1. Preheat oven to 375°F (190°C).

2. Cook lentils in vegetable broth until tender.

3. Sauté onion, garlic, carrot, zucchini, and bell pepper in olive oil. Add cooked lentils, crushed tomatoes, herbs, salt, and pepper. Simmer until thickened.

4. Mix ricotta and Parmesan (if using).

5. Spread a layer of lentil mixture in a 9x13-inch dish. Layer with noodles, ricotta mixture, and mozzarella. Repeat layers, ending with mozzarella.

6. Cover with foil and bake for 30 minutes. Remove foil and bake for another 10-15 minutes until cheese is golden. Let cool, slice, and garnish with basil.

96. Tempeh and vegetable tacos with chipotle aioli

Filling:
- 1 package tempeh, crumbled
- 2 tablespoons olive oil
- 1 bell pepper, sliced
- 1 onion, sliced
- 1 zucchini, sliced
- 1 teaspoon chili powder
- 1/2 teaspoon cumin
- Salt and pepper to taste
- Tortillas (corn or flour)

Optional Toppings:
- Sliced avocado
- Chopped cilantro
- Diced tomatoes
- Shredded lettuce
- Crumbled feta or Cotija cheese

Chipotle Aioli:
- 1/2 cup mayonnaise
- 1 tablespoon adobo sauce from canned chipotle peppers
- 1 clove garlic, minced
- 1 tablespoon lime juice
- Salt to taste

Instructions:
1. In a skillet, heat olive oil over medium heat. Add crumbled tempeh, bell pepper, onion, and zucchini. Cook until vegetables are tender and tempeh is browned.

2. Season with chili powder, cumin, salt, and pepper. Stir to combine.

3. In a small bowl, mix mayonnaise, adobo sauce, minced garlic, lime juice, and salt to make the chipotle aioli.

4. Warm tortillas in a dry skillet or microwave.

5. Fill tortillas with tempeh and vegetable mixture.

6. Drizzle chipotle aioli over the tacos.

7. Top with optional toppings like sliced avocado, chopped cilantro, diced tomatoes, shredded lettuce, or crumbled cheese.

8. Serve and enjoy your Tempeh and Vegetable Tacos with Chipotle Aioli!

97. Protein-packed peanut butter energy balls

Ingredients:
- 1 cup rolled oats
- 1/2 cup creamy peanut butter
- 1/4 cup honey or maple syrup
- 1/4 cup chocolate chips or chopped nuts (optional)
- 1/4 cup ground flaxseed or chia seeds
- 1 teaspoon vanilla extract

Instructions:

1. In a large bowl, combine rolled oats, creamy peanut butter, honey or maple syrup, chocolate chips or chopped nuts (if using), ground flaxseed or chia seeds, and vanilla extract.

2. Stir until well combined. If the mixture seems too dry, you can add a little more peanut butter or honey.

3. Using your hands, roll the mixture into balls, about 1 inch in diameter.

4. Place the energy balls on a baking sheet lined with parchment paper.

5. Refrigerate the energy balls for at least 30 minutes to firm up.

6. Once firm, transfer the energy balls to an airtight container and store them in the refrigerator for up to one week.

Enjoy your Protein-Packed Peanut Butter Energy Balls as a quick and nutritious snack to fuel your day!

98. Black bean and corn salsa with tortilla chips

Ingredients:
- 1 can (15 oz) black beans, drained and rinsed
- 1 cup corn kernels (fresh, canned, or thawed if frozen)
- 1/2 red onion, finely chopped
- 1 red bell pepper, diced
- 1 jalapeño pepper, seeded and finely chopped (optional)
- 1/4 cup chopped fresh cilantro
- Juice of 1 lime
- 1 tablespoon olive oil
- Salt and pepper to taste
- Tortilla chips, for serving

Instructions:
1. In a large bowl, combine black beans, corn kernels, finely chopped red onion, diced red bell pepper, chopped jalapeño pepper (if using), and chopped fresh cilantro.

2. Drizzle olive oil and lime juice over the mixture.

3. Season with salt and pepper to taste.

4. Gently toss everything together until well combined.

5. Cover the bowl and refrigerate the black bean and corn salsa for at least 30 minutes to allow the flavors to meld.

6. Serve the salsa chilled with tortilla chips for dipping.

Enjoy your delicious Black Bean and Corn Salsa with Tortilla Chips as a refreshing appetizer or snack!

99. Chickpea and vegetable curry with couscous

Ingredients:

For the Curry:
- 1 tablespoon olive oil
- 1 onion, diced
- 2 cloves garlic, minced
- 1 tablespoon curry powder
- 1 teaspoon ground cumin
- 1 teaspoon ground coriander
- 1/2 teaspoon ground turmeric
- 1 can (15 oz) chickpeas, drained and rinsed
- 1 can (14 oz) diced tomatoes
- 1 cup coconut milk
- 2 cups mixed vegetables (such as bell peppers, carrots, zucchini)
- Salt and pepper to taste
- Fresh cilantro for garnish (optional)

For the Couscous:
- 1 cup couscous
- 1 cup vegetable broth or water
- 1 tablespoon olive oil
- Salt to taste

Instructions:

For the Curry:

1. Heat olive oil in a large skillet over medium heat. Add diced onion and minced garlic, and sauté until softened.

2. Stir in curry powder, ground cumin, ground coriander, and ground turmeric. Cook for 1-2 minutes until fragrant.

3. Add drained and rinsed chickpeas, diced tomatoes (with juices), coconut milk, and mixed vegetables to the skillet. Season with salt and pepper to taste.

4. Bring the mixture to a simmer, then reduce heat to low. Cover and let it simmer for 15-20 minutes, or until the vegetables are tender and the curry has thickened.

5. Taste and adjust seasoning if needed. Garnish with fresh cilantro if desired.

For the Couscous:

1. In a small saucepan, bring vegetable broth or water to a boil.

2. Stir in couscous, olive oil, and salt to taste.

3. Remove from heat, cover, and let it sit for 5 minutes.

4. Fluff the couscous with a fork before serving.

Serve the chickpea and vegetable curry over the prepared couscous. Garnish with fresh cilantro if desired. Enjoy your flavorful and satisfying Chickpea and Vegetable Curry with Couscous!

100. Quinoa and vegetable sushi bowls

Ingredients:
For the Quinoa:
- 1 cup quinoa, rinsed
- 2 cups water
- 2 tablespoons rice vinegar
- 1 tablespoon sugar
- 1/2 teaspoon salt

For the Sushi Bowls:
- 2 cups cooked quinoa
- 2 cups mixed vegetables (such as cucumber, avocado, carrots, bell peppers)
- 1 cup edamame, shelled
- 4 sheets nori (seaweed), thinly sliced or crumbled
- 2 tablespoons sesame seeds
- Soy sauce or tamari, for serving
- Pickled ginger, for serving
- Wasabi, for serving
- Sriracha or spicy mayo, for serving (optional)

Instructions:
For the Quinoa:
1. In a medium saucepan, combine quinoa and water. Bring to a boil, then reduce heat to low and simmer for 15-20 minutes, or until quinoa is cooked and water is absorbed.

2. In a small bowl, mix rice vinegar, sugar, and salt until sugar and salt are dissolved.

3. Once quinoa is cooked, fluff it with a fork and stir in the rice vinegar mixture. Set aside to cool.

For the Sushi Bowls:
1. Divide cooked quinoa among serving bowls.

2. Arrange mixed vegetables and edamame on top of the quinoa.

3. Sprinkle nori slices or crumbles and sesame seeds over the vegetables.

4. Serve sushi bowls with soy sauce or tamari, pickled ginger, wasabi, and sriracha or spicy mayo (If usIng) on the side. Mix everything together before eating, if desired.

101. Greek yogurt with mixed fruit and coconut flakes

Ingredients:

- 1 cup Greek yogurt
- Assorted mixed fruits (such as berries, sliced bananas, diced mangoes, kiwi)
- 2 tablespoons coconut flakes

Instructions:

1. Spoon Greek yogurt into a serving bowl or individual cups.
2. Top with assorted mixed fruits.
3. Sprinkle coconut flakes over the yogurt and fruit.
4. Serve immediately.

Enjoy your refreshing and nutritious Greek Yogurt with Mixed Fruit and Coconut Flakes—a simple and delicious snack or breakfast option!

102. Tofu and vegetable Thai green curry

Ingredients:
- 1 tablespoon green curry paste
- 1 can (14 oz) coconut milk
- 1 block (14 oz) firm tofu, cubed
- Assorted vegetables (such as bell peppers, zucchini, carrots)
- 1 tablespoon soy sauce or tamari
- 1 tablespoon brown sugar or maple syrup
- Fresh basil or cilantro for garnish
- Cooked rice for serving

Instructions:
1. Heat green curry paste in a pan over medium heat for 1-2 minutes.

2. Pour in coconut milk and stir until combined.

3. Add cubed tofu and assorted vegetables.

4. Stir in soy sauce and brown sugar.

5. Simmer for 10-15 minutes, or until vegetables are tender and tofu is heated through.

6. Garnish with fresh basil or cilantro.

7. Serve with cooked rice.

Enjoy your flavorful Tofu and Vegetable Thai Green Curry—a quick and satisfying meal!

103. Lentil and vegetable stuffed acorn squash

Ingredients:
- 2 acorn squash
- 1 cup dry green or brown lentils, rinsed
- 2 cups vegetable broth
- 1 tablespoon olive oil
- 1 onion, diced
- 2 cloves garlic, minced
- 2 carrots, diced
- 1 zucchini, diced
- 1 bell pepper, diced
- 1 teaspoon dried thyme
- 1 teaspoon dried rosemary
- Salt and pepper to taste
- Fresh parsley for garnish

Instructions:
1. Preheat oven to 400°F (200°C).

2. Cut the acorn squash in half lengthwise and scoop out the seeds. Place them cut side down on a baking sheet lined with parchment paper. Bake for 25-30 minutes, or until squash is tender when pierced with a fork.

3. In the meantime, cook lentils in vegetable broth according to package instructions until tender.

4. In a large skillet, heat olive oil over medium heat. Add diced onion and garlic, and sauté until softened.

5. Add diced carrots, zucchini, and bell pepper to the skillet. Cook for 5-7 minutes, or until vegetables are tender.

6. Stir in cooked lentils, dried thyme, dried rosemary, salt, and pepper. Cook for an additional 2-3 minutes.

7. Once the squash is done baking, flip them over so the cut side is facing up. Fill each squash half with the lentil and vegetable mixture.

8. Return stuffed squash to the oven and bake for an additional 10-15 minutes. Garnish with fresh parsley before serving.

104. Tempeh and vegetable stir-fry with spicy peanut sauce

Ingredients:
For the Stir-Fry:
- 1 block (8 oz) tempeh, cubed
- 2 tablespoons soy sauce or tamari
- 1 tablespoon sesame oil
- 1 tablespoon olive oil
- 2 cloves garlic, minced
- 1 tablespoon grated ginger
- Assorted vegetables (such as bell peppers, broccoli, carrots, snap peas)
- Cooked rice or noodles, for serving

For the Spicy Peanut Sauce:
- 1/4 cup peanut butter
- 2 tablespoons soy sauce or tamari
- 1 tablespoon rice vinegar
- 1 tablespoon maple syrup or honey
- 1 teaspoon sriracha or chili paste (adjust to taste)
- 2-4 tablespoons water, as needed to thin the sauce

Instructions:
1. In a bowl, marinate cubed tempeh in soy sauce or tamari for 10-15 minutes.

2. In a small bowl, whisk together all ingredients for the spicy peanut sauce until smooth. Set aside.

3. Heat olive oil in a large skillet or wok over medium-high heat. Add marinated tempeh cubes and cook until browned on all sides. Remove from skillet and set aside.

4. In the same skillet, add sesame oil and sauté minced garlic and grated ginger until fragrant.

5. Add assorted vegetables to the skillet and stir-fry until they are crisp-tender.

6. Return cooked tempeh to the skillet and pour in the spicy peanut sauce. Stir well to coat everything evenly.

7. Cook for an additional 1-2 minutes, allowing the sauce to thicken slightly.

8. Serve the tempeh and vegetable stir-fry over cooked rice or noodles.

Enjoy your delicious and flavorful Tempeh and Vegetable Stir-Fry with Spicy Peanut Sauce—a satisfying and nutritious meal!

105. Protein-packed chocolate chip cookies with almond flour

Ingredients:

- 2 cups almond flour
- 1/4 cup protein powder (vanilla or chocolate flavored)
- 1/2 teaspoon baking powder
- 1/4 teaspoon salt
- 1/4 cup melted coconut oil or butter
- 1/4 cup maple syrup or honey
- 1 teaspoon vanilla extract
- 1/2 cup chocolate chips (semi-sweet or dark)

Instructions:

1. Preheat your oven to 350°F (175°C). Line a baking sheet with parchment paper.

2. In a mixing bowl, combine almond flour, protein powder, baking powder, and salt.

3. In a separate bowl, whisk together melted coconut oil or butter, maple syrup or honey, and vanilla extract until well combined.

4. Pour the wet ingredients into the dry ingredients and mix until a dough forms.

5. Fold in the chocolate chips until evenly distributed throughout the dough.

6. Scoop tablespoon-sized portions of dough and roll them into balls. Place them onto the prepared baking sheet and flatten slightly with your fingers.

7. Bake for 10-12 minutes, or until the edges are golden brown.

8. Remove from the oven and let the cookies cool on the baking sheet for a few minutes before transferring them to a wire rack to cool completely.

Enjoy your protein-packed Chocolate Chip Cookies with Almond Flour—a delicious and nutritious treat!

As you reach the end of "The Vegetarian Athlete's Guide to High-Protein Cooking: 100+ Delicious Recipes," we hope you've found inspiration, nourishment, and perhaps a few new favorite dishes along the way. Our journey through these pages has been a celebration of the incredible diversity and vitality of plant-based cuisine, showcasing the boundless possibilities for fueling your athletic pursuits with wholesome, protein-rich foods.

Whether you're a dedicated athlete, a fitness enthusiast, or simply someone looking to embrace a healthier lifestyle, we trust that the recipes and insights shared in this book have empowered you to make informed choices about your nutrition and wellness. From pre-workout snacks to post-training recovery meals, each recipe has been thoughtfully crafted to support your performance goals while delighting your taste buds.

As you continue on your journey, we encourage you to keep exploring the world of vegetarian cooking, experimenting with new ingredients, flavors, and techniques. Remember that food is not only about sustenance but also about joy, connection, and self-expression. Whether you're cooking for yourself, family, or friends, may each meal be an opportunity to nourish your body, mind, and spirit.

We extend our deepest gratitude to you for joining us on this culinary adventure. Your enthusiasm, curiosity, and dedication to your health inspire us to continue sharing the transformative power of plant-based eating. As you savor the final pages of this book, know that your journey towards peak performance and vibrant well-being is just beginning.

Here's to a future filled with vitality, strength, and countless delicious meals enjoyed in the company of those you love. Cheers to your health, happiness, and continued success as a vegetarian athlete. Keep cooking, keep moving, and keep thriving!

With warmest wishes and gratitude,

Gustav Henning